AROMATHERAPY ANSWERS

Your Practical Guide to Common Ailments

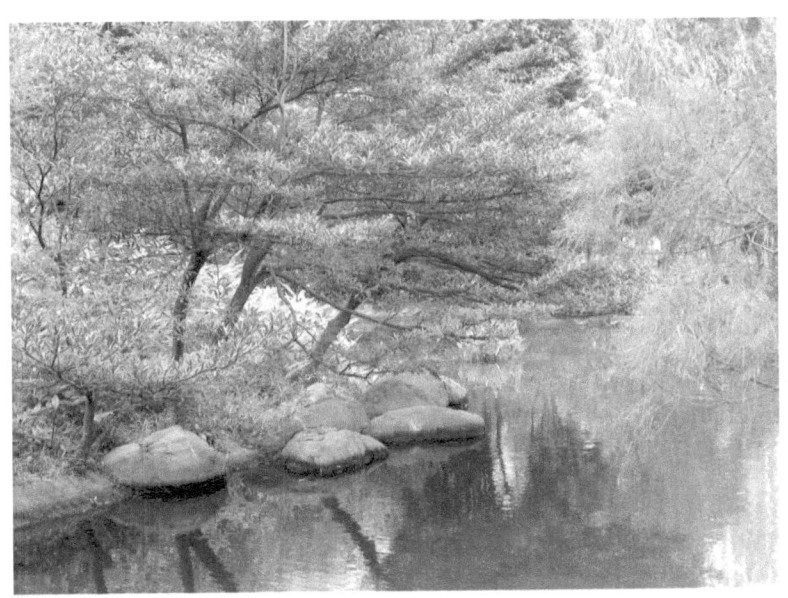

By

Judith Fitzsimmons
with Paula M. Bousquet

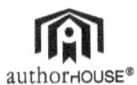

authorHOUSE®

AuthorHouse™
1663 Liberty Drive
Bloomington, IN 47403
www.authorhouse.com
Phone: 1-800-839-8640

Published by AuthorHouse 11/25/2014

ISBN: 978-1-4208-1141-4 (sc)

Library of Congress Control Number: 2004099088

Any people depicted in stock imagery provided by Thinkstock are models, and such images are being used for illustrative purposes only. Certain stock imagery © Thinkstock.

This book is printed on acid-free paper.

Book Credits

Sanjay Pindiyath and Susan Evilla Pindiyath took all photographs. For a special treat, visit some more of their work at http://www.morguefile.com/forum_testing/profile.php?username=pindiyath100&mode=viewprofile.

Front Cover Creative Inspiration by Kevin M. Harkness.

Disclaimer

This book was designed and written to provide information about and methods of use of the subject matter covered. This information is not intended to be used to treat, diagnose, or prescribe, and is in no way to be considered as a substitute for consultation with a duly licensed health care professional.

Dedication

To my mother, Marie Mazzeo Fitzsimmons, who lives forever, if only in my heart. To my daughter, Chelsea Marie Gunn, whom I want to make as proud of me as I am of her. And to Mark, my gift, my tomorrow.

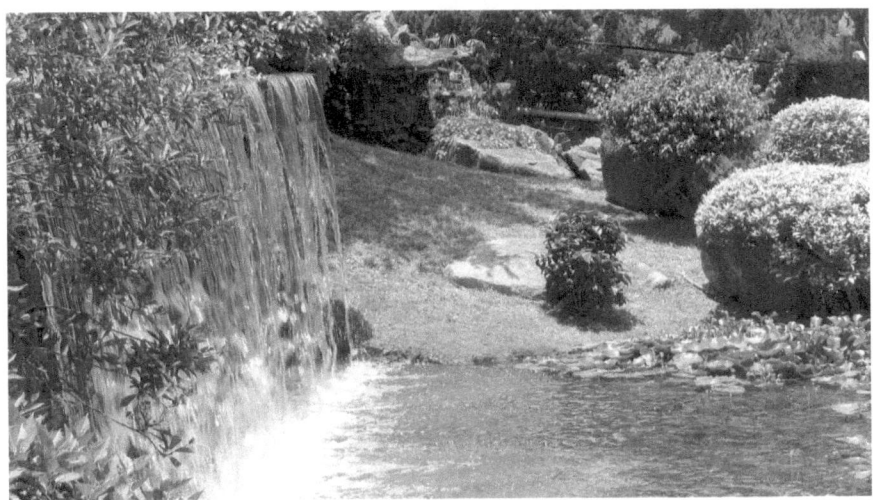

Acknowledgements

Whenever I read another author's acknowledgements, I always think, "Gosh, they are thanking just about everyone they know, what's up with that?" And now, here I sit thinking about the people who were involved in getting *Aromatherapy Answers* to you and I understand, so bear with me.

Thanks to Paula M. Bousquet who always kept the reader at the forefront. To MJ Plaster whose constructive criticism made this book even better, and whose humor kept me sane. To Ellen Simes who always makes me sound so wonderful and is more than wonderful herself. To Cynthia Nishimura for, well first of all, for twenty-four years of honest, loving friendship, and for her clarity and focus towards the details of this book. To Penny Gauder whom you readers should thank because her questions got most of your questions answered.

There are not enough words of respect and appreciation that I can give to my photographers, Sanjay Pindiyath and Susan Evilla Pindiyath. They not only worked with our time difference (they live in Hong Kong and I live in Tennessee), but they also shared their passion, gift, and talent with me through the photographs you see throughout this book. For a special treat, visit some more of their work at http://www.morguefile.com/forum testing/profile.php?username=pindiyath100&mode=viewprofile.

To my other readers who I only met through their dedication to making this book as useful and informative as it is, including Amy L. Taylor, Melissa J. Hayes, and Tammy Smith – I should curse you for the extra work, but since it made the book that much better for the readers, I have to say a heartfelt thanks.

To Carol Harkness, I'm so glad that a penny war led to such an adventure. To her son, Kevin Harkness, keep up the creative work!

To my family and friends who I practically ignored this past year just so I could keep writing – thanks for your patience and understanding. To my aromatherapy clients who have shared their lives with me, and allowed me to assist them in managing their health through natural solutions. And to Chelsea and Mark who endured countless burned meals, washer-dyed clothing, and occasional grumpiness – can we blame it all on the book?

Table of Contents

Introduction

A journey that started 13 years ago has evolved into a way of life for me, my family and friends, and many of my clients. During the past six years, through my business, Aromatherapy Solutions, I have worked with hundreds of people to help them learn about the healthy and practical uses of essential oils. By incorporating aromatherapy into their lives, I have witnessed countless people move away from synthetic and harmful products towards a more natural and balanced lifestyle. During a discussion one particular client said, "You should put all of the answers to the questions people have asked you over the years into a book." And so I have. The "Question and Answer" section provides an overview to aromatherapy by answering the most frequently asked questions I have heard over the years.

Taking it a step further, I decided to extend the gift of knowledge and experience by making it easy for you to introduce aromatherapy into your life. The rest of the book provides several practical solutions for everyday ailments. My goal was to provide thought-provoking information in a friendly, informative, and personal way. It is my hope that this book will help you on your exploration of aromatherapy and help you to start realizing the value and benefit of these natural gifts.

– Judi

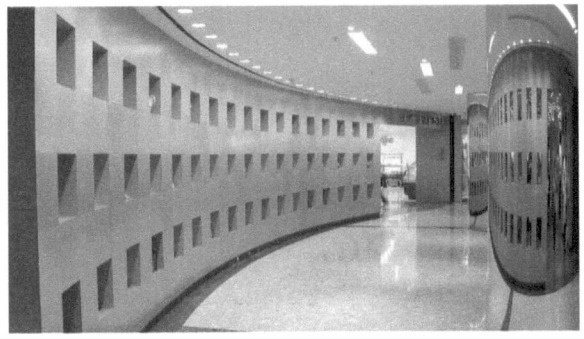

Questions and Answers

In all things of nature there is something of the marvelous.

Aristotle

What is Aromatherapy?

Aromatherapy is the use of natural plant essences to create a positive effect on your health and enhance your natural beauty. Aromatherapists have been using essential oils since the beginning of time – really the beginning of time. Essential oils are extracted from plants. Some people consider them to be the plant's blood stream because they contain all the chemicals, oxygen, hormones, and nutrients that sustain the plant.

How do they get essential oils from plants?

Essential oils are extracted from various parts of the plant. For example, the citrus essential oils, such as orange, lemon, and grapefruit, are extracted from the peel. When people think about essential oils, they think they come from the flower of the plant. Some essential oils, such as Lavender and Chamomile, do come from the flower. In other cases, the essential oil can be extracted from many parts of the plant, for example, from the berries of the Juniper plant, or from the bark of the Cedar tree.

In extracting these essential oils from the various parts of the plants, we are taking the essence of the plant, including its nutrients and chemicals; thus the name essential oils. These essential components also contain chemical compounds that are valuable in healing.

Did you just say chemical?

How can I talk about essential oils being natural and still have chemical composition and properties? We, as consumers, may associate chemicals with synthetic, and often harmful, chemicals, but if you remember back to high school chemistry class, chemicals are not necessarily synthetic.

How can smelling something heal you?

I prefer to call Aromatherapy, Essential Oil Therapy because it is the chemical composition of the essential oils that heal. No matter how much you smell an aromatherapy blend, that won't help lower back pain. But when you mix several oils that have analgesic and anti-inflammatory properties, and massage that blend on your back, you are going to get some great results.

How do essential oils work?

Like many drugs, essential oils work by sending chemicals into the blood stream where the healing properties can travel through the body. One of the advantages aromatherapy has over pharmaceuticals is that you do not have to ingest essential oils. As such, the valuable chemicals in the essential oils are not diluted by stomach enzymes and are not processed through your liver and/or kidney before they start working.

How do I use essential oils?

Aromatherapy Answers is a recipe book that uses three predominant methods of using essential oils:

Dark Glass Container

Several recipes instruct you to mix all of the essential oils together in a dark glass container. From there, I might suggest that you use a portion of the combined essential oils in water and another portion in lotion or oil. In rare cases, such as Acne, I suggest that you apply the essential oils directly.

The reason you are to mix the essential oils together in a dark glass container are (a) essential oils last longer if they are not exposed to light and the dark glass helps, and (b) essential oils are so concentrated that if you use a non-glass container, they may actually "melt" plastic or rubber and destroy your blend.

Lotion or Oil-Based

Because essential oils are so concentrated, you should dilute them in a "carrier." The role of the carrier is to carry the essential oils safely into the body. The carrier may be a lotion, cream, oil, or even water. See the "Carriers" chapter for details.

Water-Based

Many recipes suggest that you add the essential oils to water. In today's world, we are often anxious about the quality of our water. Having said that let me also say that I am a frugal person. You do not have to use distilled water, but filtered water is recommended. If you use tap water, be sure to boil it first, then let it cool to room temperature before mixing with essential oils.

What do scientists believe about essential oils?

The medical and scientific communities have proven that essential oils are the most oxygen-producing entities known to mankind. They have also proven that disease cannot live within an oxygen-rich environment. These professionals are now exploring what combination of essential oils can be used to offset, not only everyday illness, but also the more significant diseases that punish our world.

How quickly do essential oils start working?

Essential oils start working right away. Five seconds after you apply essential oils, they begin to affect every cell in your body. Within 21 seconds they can affect EVERY cell. Twenty-one minutes later they reach their peak of effectiveness. 2 ½ hours later there is no more chemical residue in your body. However, the therapeutic effect can last for months.

With this said, you have to understand that it is going to take some blends minutes, hours, days, weeks, and even months before you get the cumulative benefit of the blend. There are a couple of reasons that it takes some blends longer to work than others including:

- Access – how close to the surface of the skin is the area you are trying to treat? For example, a cut or scrape is going to respond more quickly than cellulite because the cut is closer to the surface of the skin where you are applying the essential oil blend.

- Complexity – how complex is the area you are treating? For example, a sinus pocket looks like a large kidney bean (not too complex), so it will respond more quickly than arthritis where you are dealing with bone, joint, tendon, cartilage, and muscle (more complex).

- Length of time – how long have you had the problem? Children respond more quickly to essential oil blends than adults.

- Continuation – are you continuing to damage the area you are treating? This frequently happens with carpal tunnel, sprains, or any other ailment where you are continuing to aggravate the injury.

So if the instructions in some blends suggest that you use the blend for several weeks or months, now you know why.

Are all essential oils safe for everyone to use?

No, as is true with any chemical, you want to be aware of any contraindications (warnings and precautions) to make sure that the essential oil is safe for you. See the "Essential Oil Chart" in the Appendix for safety information. Also on the issue of safety, be sure to use the essential oils as directed.

Another issue of safety deals with chemical interactions (between prescribed medications and essential oils, or even when using multiple essential oil blends at the same time). If you are taking a prescribed medication, be sure to check with your doctor about other chemicals you should avoid when taking this medication. Many over-the-counter medications have fewer ingredients that could negatively interact with other chemicals; that's why they are over the counter. But you would still want to read the box for any cautions or warnings, and not use any other chemical that could counteract what you are treating.

How many ailments can I treat at one time?

Being the pragmatic person that I am, I try to control as many variables when I am trying to remedy something. For example, if I am treating a person for razor burn, there are several natural things they can do, such as reducing the pressure they apply while shaving, not using products that contain synthetic fragrances, dyes, and alcohol, and shaving in the direction of the hair growth. I usually suggest that they try these natural solutions first to see if it improves their condition. If they are still having trouble, then we try the essential oil blends. We can then measure the effectiveness of the blend because it is now the only thing that was different about their usual routine – the results can be credited directly to the essential oils.

If you have a list of ailments you want to treat, I would suggest that as long as the treatment for one ailment does not interfere with the treatment of another ailment, then get yourself healthy quickly. For example, the natural suggestions and essential oil blends for cellulite would have no benefit for sinus problems, so go ahead and treat cellulite and sinus at the same time. However, the natural suggestions and essential oil blends for arthritis in the knee may influence the essential oil blends for a strained leg muscle. Having said that, most of my clients say, "I don't really see the need to know exactly what worked as long as it works." I guess that is just the practical, no-nonsense side of me.

Will all blends work for me?

No. Every person is different so some blends will work very well for some people and not as well for others. Think about the number of sinus and allergy products (prescribed and over-the-counter) on the market today. If only one of those products worked on ALL people, we would only have one product on the market. Pharmaceutical companies and aromatherapists make several different chemical combinations to treat the same ailment in an effort to have the right chemical combination for each person. Therefore, if one of the blends doesn't seem to be working as expected, try a different one.

Can I combine blends or double the amount of essential oils in a blend?

Throughout the book, you will see that I suggest one blend at the onset of an ailment, and then as you improve, I suggest a different blend. So, you might wonder if you can combine those blends and just use that instead. The answer is no because each blend is formulated for specific conditions.

You also need to understand that essential oils are extremely concentrated and, as such, should not be over used. More is not better when it comes to essential oils. Therefore, I do not suggest that you increase the number of drops in any of these blends.

Still not sure?

Like you, many people are skeptical when they first think about using essential oil solutions for physical, mental, or emotional ailments. But they examined aromatherapy because a) they were not getting the desired results from conventional medicines, b) they were taking significant synthetic drugs that were giving them undesirable side effects, c) they were looking for a solution that worked in harmony with their body's natural ability to heal itself, and (d) they were looking for a more cost-effective solution, especially if the ailment they were treating will need ongoing support, such as arthritis.

Where can I buy essential oils?

At the back of the book is an order form from which you can order therapeutic grade, high quality essential oils from me. Be sure to look at the Essential Oil Chart to learn about the essential oils and do not purchase any oils that are contraindicated for you. Also, citrus oils oxidize quickly which means they evaporate quickly, and resin-based oils can get thick and gooey quickly, so keep that in mind when ordering.

What About Vaporizers?

The idea of running a vaporizer scares a lot of people because they believe it can cause mold. If you are running a warm-mist vaporizer for an extended period of time, you can encourage mold. Therefore, I suggest a cool-mist vaporizer to avoid the production of mold while getting the benefits from increased hydration.

From the moment we close the windows and turn on the heat in the fall, I run my cool-mist vaporizer every night. Depending on what I am trying to prevent, I use different essential oils in the vaporizer. Sometimes, I simply run straight water. The cool mist keeps the hydration in your home so that your nasal passages stay lubricated. I always look for the least expensive vaporizer that is just a plain plastic tub with a spinning device inside. I don't want cup holders, filters, or pads. I fill the plain tub with water, add the oils directly, and I'm ready to go. You should clean your vaporizer every week. Use the Antiseptic Spray blend from the "Infection" chapter to clean out the vaporizer. Be sure to clean the spinning device to remove any excess essential oils.

Note: Inhalation via cool mist is NOT recommended for individuals who suffer with asthma.

Why use Aromatherapy?

Some people will start using essential oils because they want to take care of their family, even their pets, using natural products. Other people just love the idea that it makes financial sense. For just pennies, you can replace your basic skin care products, cleaning supplies, and many of your medications with aromatherapy solutions that are just as effective.

How do I get started with Aromatherapy?

With all of the aromatherapy-related products you see in department stores, pharmacies, and other retail stores, you would think it would be easy to get started with aromatherapy. Unfortunately, about 90% of the products that you see on the market today do not contain one drop of essential oil. Therefore, these are not aromatherapy products at all, but rather products that smell nice.

The best way to get started with aromatherapy is to learn about it. That is what this book is intended to do — help you learn about essential oils, their chemical properties, how to make formulations, and how to successfully use them in your daily life.

Also, feel free to visit my website www.aromatherapysolutions.com on which you can find many articles and more useful information.

Before You Begin

"There is no such thing as can't, only won't."

Jan Ashford

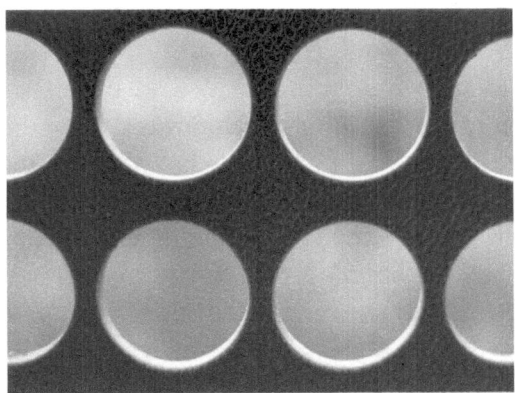

If you opened the book directly to this page, then you are a lot like me, wanting to get into the heart of things. We are the type of people who believe that there is no such thing as can't, so we want to prove that we can. However, we also know that we have to do our research so I strongly suggest that you read the "Introduction" chapter. It provides a great deal of information that will make your experience with using essential oils more successful. At least read the answers in the "Introduction" chapter to these questions so that you can set realistic expectations for using essential oils:

How do essential oils work?

Will all blends work for me?

How quickly do essential oils start working?

The remaining chapters are arranged by category for quick reference. Within each category, the ailments are listed alphabetically so you can easily find the ailment you want to explore. You can also use the Table of Contents for a concise view of the ailments. Be sure to use the Index if something you are interested in has a slightly different name; for example, I called indigestion, Indigestion, but if you are looking for gastrointestinal ailment, you will find that in the Index.

The Appendix includes two very useful chapters on properties of carrier oils and an essential oil chart the contains valuable information about the ailments you can treat with essential oils and any cautions you should be aware of.

Finally, I have included a form, which you can use to purchase quality, therapeutic essential oils at very reasonable rates. I would suggest that you go through the book and mark the list of ailments you are interesting in exploring. Then, create a list of the essential oils for those blends and base your order on your current needs. Since the essential oils have a shelf life of about 18 months, do not order an oil that you are not going to use within that time frame.

For additional information about essential oils, some additional free recipes, or to contact me, please feel free to visit www.aromatherapysolutions.com.

Aches & Pains

How do you apply essential oils to aches and pains?

To treat aches and pains, including bruises, muscle aches, or sprains anywhere on your body, apply the essential oil blends in a straight upward motion; do not use circular motions. The reason for this is that you want to work in the same direction as your body. If you rub in a circular motion, you are actually constricting the parts of your body that you are trying to treat versus working with the flow of your internal body structure. Think about putting an elastic band in your hand and imagine that the elastic band is your muscle. If you rub the elastic band in a circular motion, it becomes this twisted little ball or knot. That is what is happening to your muscles if you apply blends in a circular motion; obviously, not a healthy result. This is one time when the expression, "Go with the flow" really applies.

The remainder of this section deals with:

- Ankle Sprain

- Arthritis (osteo and rheumatoid)

- Back Pain

- Carpal Tunnel Syndrome

- Muscle Aches and Pains (bruised/cramped/sprain/strain)

- Neck Sprain

- Pain Relief

- Tendonitis

Ankle Sprain

"If you are distressed by anything external, the pain is not due to the thing itself but to your own estimate of it; and this you have the power to revoke at any moment."

Marcus Aurelius

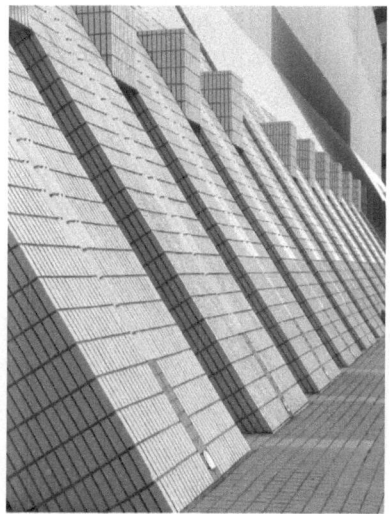

Marcus Aurelius Antoninus is regarded as one of the greatest emperors in Roman history, an intelligent philosopher, and a leader driven to find peace. His quotation reflects much of what he was and can inspire us as we deal with external pain in our life. I'm sure he would have been relieved to use some natural solutions and practical assistance for relieving sprains.

Sprain refers to damage or tearing of ligaments. When excessive force is applied to a joint, the ligaments that hold the bones together may be torn or damaged — the result is a sprain. Its seriousness depends on how badly the ligaments are torn. Any joint can be sprained, but the most frequently injured joints are the ankle, knee, and finger.

Children under age eight are less likely to have sprains than are older people. Children's ligaments are tighter, and their bones are more apt to break before a ligament tears. People who are active in sports suffer more strains and sprains than less active people.

There are three grades of sprains:

- Grade I sprains are mild injuries where there is no tearing of the ligament and no joint function is lost. There may be tenderness and slight swelling.

- With a Grade II sprain there is obvious swelling, extensive bruising, pain, and it is hard to bear weight.

- Grade III sprains are caused by complete tearing of the ligament where there is severe pain, loss of joint function, widespread swelling and bruising, and you cannot bear weight.

Grade I sprains can be treated at home. Basic first aid for sprains consists of RICE: Rest, Ice for 48 hours, Compression (wrapping in an elastic bandage), and Elevation of the sprain above the level of the heart. Over-the-counter pain medication can be taken for pain. People with grade II and grade III sprains should consult a physician. If the sprain is in the ankle or knee, you may need to use crutches until the sprains have healed enough to bear weight. Occasionally, physical therapy or home exercises are needed to restore the strength and flexibility of the joint. Grade III sprains usually need to be immobilized in a cast for several weeks to see if the sprain heals.

Many times, sprains and strains can be prevented by warming-up before exercising, using proper lifting techniques, wearing properly fitting shoes, and taping or bracing the joint.

Essential Oil Blends

Sprains react very well to these essential oils: Black Pepper, Chamomile, Clove, Cypress, Eucalyptus, Ginger, Lavender, Marjoram, Nutmeg, Peppermint, Pine, Rosemary, Thyme, and Vetiver. Refer to the "Essential Oil Chart" for contraindications, warnings, or cautions about using essential oils.

When you first sprain your ankle — or any other muscle/joint — the Ankle Sprain Relief blend is great for reducing the pain. However, keep in mind that pain reminds you to not overdo or shorten the healing process, so use the blend just enough to relieve the significant pain.

I don't think we really appreciate how valuable our ankles are until we sprain them. We stretch our leg muscles before and after we exercise, we soak our feet, and we even do pedicures, but we often neglect our precious ankles.

To treat bruises, muscle aches, or sprains anywhere on your body, apply the essential oil blends in a straight upward motion; see the "Aches & Pains" section for details.

Ankle Sprain Relief

13 drops Clove

15 drops Ginger

10 drops Lavender

20 drops Nutmeg

> Mix all the oils together in a dark glass container. For the first 48 hours, apply a cold compress to the affected area as often as possible, up to 3 times per hour. Place 3 drops of the essential oil mixture onto the cold wet cloth before each application. Keep the compress on the affected area until the cloth reaches room temperature. Elevate the foot.
>
> After 48 hours, add the remainder of the essential oil mixture to 2 ounces of base lotion or 2 tablespoons carrier oil (any oil listed in the "Carrier Oils" chapter). Apply a small amount of the blend to the area of injury and the areas immediately above and below the site of injury. Apply the blend 4 to 6 times a day for the first 5 – 7 days until the pain subsides.

When the pain has eased, you may want to switch to the Ankle Sprain Soother blend because Eucalyptus promotes the health of red and white blood cells, which facilitates healing. The blend also contains pain-relieving oils.

Ankle Sprain Soother

10 drops Cypress

15 drops Eucalyptus

10 drops Lavender

13 drops Peppermint

Add the essential oils to 4 ounces of base lotion or 4 tablespoons carrier oil (any oil listed in the "Carrier Oils" chapter). Apply a small amount of the blend to the area of injury and the areas immediately above and below the site of injury. Apply the blend 4 to 6 times a day for the first 5 – 7 days and then reduce to twice daily until your ankle feels strong and totally free of pain.

Arthritis

"I don't deserve this award, but I have arthritis and I don't deserve that either."

Jack Benny

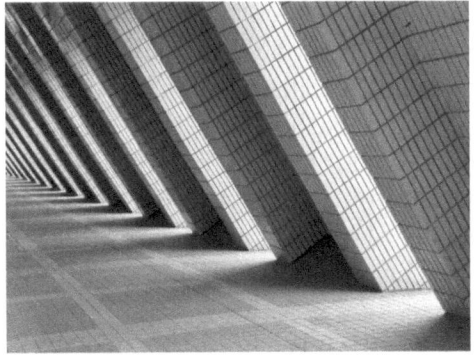

Jack Benny's humor has brought great joy to millions of people for decades. However, there is nothing humorous about arthritis. Fortunately, much medical and scientific research continues towards better understanding and finding successful treatments for arthritis. Until the glorious day arrives when there is a cure, investigate alternatives to treating your pain and other symptoms.

Arthritis causes pain and swelling in your joints. Joints are places where two bones meet, such as your elbow or knee. Over time, arthritic joints can become severely damaged. Symptoms of arthritis include: swelling in one or more joints, stiffness around the joints that lasts for at least 1 hour after getting up, constant or recurring pain or tenderness in a joint, difficulty using or moving a joint normally, and warmth and redness in a joint.

There are several kinds of arthritis; the two most common are rheumatoid arthritis and osteoarthritis. Osteoarthritis is the most common form of arthritis, affecting an estimated 21 million adults in the United States. This is the form that usually comes with age and most often affects cartilage, which is the tissue that cushions the ends of bones within the joints in your fingers, knees, and hips. Sometimes osteoarthritis follows an injury to a joint. For example, a young person hurts his knee badly playing sports. Years after the knee has apparently healed, he might get arthritis in his knee joint.

Rheumatoid arthritis is an inflammatory disease of the synovium, or lining of the joint, which results in pain, stiffness, swelling, joint damage, and loss of function of the joints. Inflammation most often affects joints of the hands and feet and tends to be symmetrical (occurring equally on both sides of the body). This symmetry helps distinguish rheumatoid arthritis from other forms of arthritis. About 1 percent of the U.S. population has rheumatoid arthritis.

While there is no cure for arthritis, there are treatments that you can discuss with your doctor, including rest and relaxation, exercise, proper diet, medication, and instruction about the proper use of joints and ways to conserve energy. Other treatments include pain relief methods and assistive devices, such as splints or braces. In severe cases, surgery may be suggested.

Things that you can do to help yourself are: keep your weight down, exercise, keep warm by taking a warm shower in the morning and dressing warmly in winter. Make sure you have the proper amount of calcium, vitamin C, and vitamin E in your diet.

Essential Oil Blends

Essential oils that can help relieve arthritis pain are the following:

- Black Pepper, Carrot, Cedarwood, Chamomile (both German and Roman), Clove, Eucalyptus, Ginger, Peppermint, Pine, Rosemary, Thyme, Vetiver, and Yarrow have good pain relieving properties and promote healing.

- Birch, Juniper, Marjoram, Nutmeg, Sage, and Spruce draw out pain.

Refer to the "Essential Oil Chart" for contraindications, warnings, or cautions about using essential oils.

I have arthritis in my knee and yet I still want to coach my daughter's soccer and softball teams, so I use the blends described here and find that water aerobics and stretching exercises make it possible for me to do the things I enjoy with little or no pain.

See the "Aches & Pains" section for information about how to apply blends to joint pain and how quickly essential oil blends work.

The Arthritis Pain Relief blend contains a few more pain-relieving essential oils than the other blends. You might want to use this blend first to ease pain. With all essential oils blends, but especially the pain relief blends, you want to use a small amount of the blend as often as possible for the first few days. More frequent application is much more effective than overdoing a couple of applications a day.

Arthritis (osteo) Pain Relief

4 drops Black Pepper

8 drops Chamomile

6 drops Cypress

6 drops Ginger

4 drops Juniper

4 drops Peppermint

4 drops Rosemary

> There is no medical or alternative cure for osteoarthritis — the blend is intended to help alleviate the associated pain.
>
> Add all essential oils to 2 ounces of base lotion or 2 tablespoons of carrier oil (any oil listed in the "Carrier Oils" chapter). Apply a small amount of the blend to the affected area and the areas immediately above and below the affected area. Apply the blend 4 to 6 times a day for at least two weeks until the pain subsides.
>
> If the pain does not subside after two weeks, continue to apply the blend 4 to 6 times daily for up to 6 weeks. Individual progress with arthritis varies.

When the pain has eased, you may want to switch to the Arthritis Assistance blend because Eucalyptus promotes the health of red and white blood cells thus facilitating healing. The blend also contains pain-relieving oils.

Arthritis (osteo) Assistance

4 drops Eucalyptus

6 drops Ginger

8 drops Lavender

4 drops Marjoram

4 drops Rosemary

4 drops Spruce

> There is no medical or alternative cure for osteoarthritis, so the blend is intended to help alleviate the associated pain.
>
> Add all essential oils to 2 ounces of base lotion or 2 tablespoons of carrier oil (any oil listed in the "Carrier Oils" chapter). Apply a small amount of the blend to the affected area and the areas immediately above and below the affected area. Apply the blend 4 to 6 times a day for at least two weeks until the pain subsides.
>
> If the pain does not subside after two weeks, continue to apply the blend 4 to 6 times daily for up to 6 weeks. Individual progress with arthritis varies.

All three of the Rheumatoid Arthritis blends contain strong pain-relieving properties. They also contain oils that have the ability to draw deep-seated pain out. You can make your selection based on which essential oils you already have or use the less expensive essential oils.

Arthritis (rheumatoid) Pain Reliever

8 drops Chamomile

6 drops Cypress

6 drops Ginger

4 drops Peppermint

4 drops Rosemary

4 drops Spruce

> Add all essential oils to 2 ounces of base lotion or 2 tablespoons of carrier oil (any oil listed in the "Carrier Oils" chapter). Apply a small amount of the blend to the affected area and the areas immediately above and below the affected area. Apply the blend 4 to 6 times a day for at least two weeks until the pain subsides.

> If the pain does not subside after two weeks, continue to apply the blend 4 to 6 times daily for up to 6 weeks. Individual progress with arthritis varies.

It is very important to support the entire area that is affected by the arthritis, so be sure to apply the blend above and below the area as well.

Arthritis (rheumatoid) Pain Soother

6 drops Black Pepper

6 drops Ginger

4 drops Lavender

8 drops Marjoram

4 drops Peppermint

4 drops Vetiver

> Add all essential oils to 2 ounces of base lotion or 2 tablespoons of carrier oil (any oil listed in the "Carrier Oils" chapter). Apply a small amount of the blend to the affected area and the areas immediately above and below the affected area. Apply the blend 4 to 6 times a day for at least two weeks until the pain subsides.

> If the pain does not subside after two weeks, continue to apply the blend 4 to 6 times daily for up to 6 weeks. Individual progress with arthritis varies.

One pain management theory suggests that the body requires symmetrical treatment. What this means is that if you are suffering from arthritis in your left knee, you should treat the right knee as well.

I have been treating both of my knees even though the pain is more significant in one. I guess I just figured if I had arthritis in one knee, I would get it in the other knee, so some preventative pain relief is appreciated.

Arthritis (rheumatoid) Pain Management

2 drops Chamomile

8 drops Clove

12 drops Ginger

10 drops Nutmeg

Add all essential oils to 2 ounces of base lotion or 2 tablespoons of carrier oil (any oil listed in the "Carrier Oils" chapter). Apply a small amount of the blend to the affected area and the areas immediately above and below the affected area. Apply the blend 4 to 6 times a day for at least two weeks until the pain subsides.

If the pain does not subside after two weeks, continue to apply the blend 4 to 6 times daily for up to 6 weeks. Individual progress with arthritis varies.

Back Pain

"The art of life is the art of avoiding pain."

Thomas Jefferson

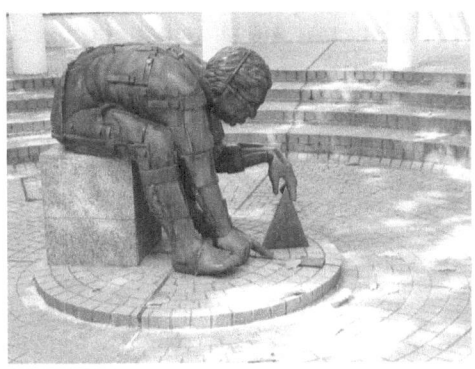

We can certainly agree with Thomas Jefferson about trying to avoid pain. We all know that in today's rush and tumble world it is often very difficult to avoid pain. I have worked with several people who not only have back pain, but also have a job that requires activities that may exacerbate the pain. There is much we can do to ease back pain: using support appliances, stretching, exercising, aromatherapy, and more. Investigate your options so you can treat pain whenever you can't avoid it.

The cause of back pain can be as simple as lifting something the wrong way, overexerting a muscle, or trauma due to illness or injury. There are some common behaviors that can contribute to back pain. These include sitting for extended periods of time — especially in a poorly designed chair, sleeping on a mattress that doesn't offer proper support, carrying more weight than you should, untreated foot problems, and wearing improper shoes. In addition to keeping an eye on these behaviors, you can help keep your back pain free by warming up before any activity, exercising regularly, lifting objects properly, and dealing effectively with stress.

Sometimes, diagnosing and treating back pain can be a complex matter that requires professional attention, so if you have persistent back pain of an undetermined origin, consult your physician.

For back pain caused by overextended muscles or muscle strain, for the first 48 hours you may want to apply ice to slow down inflammation and provide temporary pain relief. After 48 hours, heat may be more beneficial. For some people, alternating heat with cold application provides the most pain relief. There is no exact prescription for ice and heat application. Many physicians and physical therapists recommend trying different forms of heat and cold application to see which approach provides the most pain relief.

Essential Oil Blends

For their pain relieving properties and to promote healing, consider Cedarwood, Chamomile (both German and Roman), Eucalyptus, Ginger, Peppermint, Pine, Rosemary, Thyme, or Vetiver. To draw out the pain try Basil, Lemongrass, Marjoram, Nutmeg, Sage, or Spruce. Refer to the "Essential Oil Chart" for contraindications, warnings, or cautions about using essential oils.

When you first injure your back or any other muscle, the Back Pain Relief blend is great for reducing the pain. Keep in mind that pain reminds you not to overdo or shorten the healing process, so use this blend just enough to relieve the significant pain.

To treat bruises, muscle aches, or sprains anywhere on your body, apply the essential oil blends in a straight upward motion; see the "Aches & Pains" section for details.

My fiancé was lifting heavy materials for a building project and would not put the project on hold until his back healed. He used the Back Pain Relief and finished the project.

Back Pain Relief

15 drops Chamomile

13 drops Clary Sage

15 drops Lavender

10 drops Peppermint

> Mix all the oils together in a dark glass container. For the first 48 hours, apply a cold compress to the affected area as often as possible, up to 3 times per hour. Place 3 drops of the blend onto the cold wet cloth prior to each application. Keep the compress on the affected area until the cloth reaches room temperature.
>
> After 48 hours, add the remainder of the essential oils to 2 ounces of base lotion or 2 tablespoons carrier oil (any oil listed in the "Carrier Oils" chapter). Apply a small amount of the blend to the area of injury and the areas immediately above and below the site of injury. Apply the blend 4 to 6 times a day for the first 5 – 7 days until the pain subsides.

When the pain has eased, you may want to switch to the Back Pain Soother blend. The Eucalyptus promotes the health of red and white blood cells, which facilitates healing. This blend also contains pain-relieving oils.

Back Pain Soother

10 drops Cypress

15 drops Eucalyptus

15 drops Lavender

15 drops Marjoram

10 drops Peppermint

> Add all the oils to 2 ounces of base lotion or 2 tablespoons carrier oil (any oil listed in the "Carrier Oils" chapter). Apply a small amount of the blend to the area of injury and the areas immediately above and below the site of injury. Apply the blend 4 to 6 times a day for the first 5 – 7 days until the pain subsides.

Use the Back Pain Support blend after your back has healed to continue providing support to the large muscles.

Back Pain Support

10 drops Eucalyptus

10 drops Peppermint

10 drops Rosemary

> Mix all oils together. Use in any of these ways:
>
> Put 10 drops in 2 tablespoons of carrier oil and massage the affected area. The ideal time to do this is after a warm bath and before bedtime.
>
> Put 8 drops in a bath. Relax your cares away while you deep soak the strain from your muscles.

Carpal Tunnel Syndrome

"When you do the common things in life in an uncommon way, you will command the attention of the world."

George Washington Carver

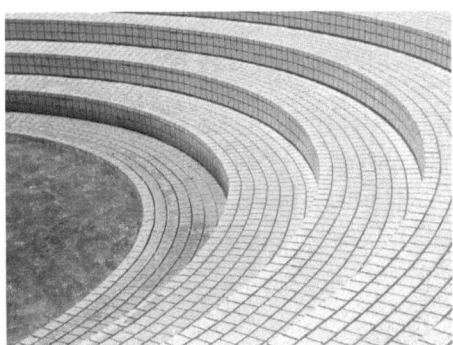

With this common but misunderstood ailment, healing in an uncommon way is quite effective. While George Washington Carver was not talking about carpal tunnel syndrome, performing common activities to an uncommon degree will get your attention. Imagine a waiter carrying heavy trays during an 8-hour shift or a beautician using scissors for 6 to 8 hours a day — common things done to an uncommon degree. Let aromatherapy support your body so that it can maintain its health.

You can find a lot of detailed and scientific information about carpal tunnel syndrome, but I am going to give you just the introduction. Carpal Tunnel Syndrome is an extremely common, as well as a very misunderstood, condition. If you have compressed the median nerve in your hand, you have Carpal Tunnel Syndrome. The compression of the nerve is the result of inflammation.

Symptoms include numbness and tingling in the hand – this often begins at night — with pain and weakness in the hand — particularly in the thumb. Carpal Tunnel Syndrome often coincides with related conditions such as tendonitis in the fingers or in the wrist.

It is believed that Carpal Tunnel Syndrome can be triggered by a repetitive activity that causes discomfort to the hands and wrist, such as carrying heavy objects or data entry work. It seems to occur most often in middle-aged women, often perimenopausal, and woman in their third trimester of pregnancy.

The treatment for Carpal Tunnel Syndrome is directed at decreasing the inflammation of the tendons. Night splints (to ease the pressure on the wrist) and medicinal drugs to reduce inflammation are the most common treatment.

Essential Oil Blends

Essential oils that can help promote nerve health and circulation are: Basil, Cypress, Eucalyptus, Lavender, Lemongrass, Marjoram, and Peppermint. Refer to the "Essential Oil Chart" for contraindications, warnings, or cautions about using essential oils.

Some of the first symptoms of carpal tunnel are tightness in the veins and muscles followed by tingling in the fingers and throbbing pain. To reduce the swelling and relieve the pain, use the Carpal Tunnel Relief blend.

I started studying aromatherapy when I was pregnant and the timing couldn't have been better, because instead of going for surgery for the carpal tunnel symptoms I experienced in my third trimester, I used aromatherapy.

See the "Aches & Pains" section for information about how to apply essential oil blends to an injury such as carpal tunnel and how long it may take for you to receive pain relief.

Carpal Tunnel Relief

10 drops Eucalyptus

10 drops Lavender

10 drops Marjoram

2 drops Peppermint

> Add all essential oils to 2 ounces of base lotion or 2 tablespoons of of carrier oil (any oil listed in the "Carrier Oils" chapter). Apply a small amount of the blend to the affected area and the areas immediately above and below the affected area. Apply the blend 4 to 6 times a day for at least two weeks until the pain subsides.

> If the pain does not subside after two weeks, continue to apply the blend 4 to 6 times daily for up to 6 weeks. Individual progress with carpal tunnel varies.

Most or my working day is spent on a keyboard, so I use the Carpal Tunnel Soother on a regular basis to prevent any symptoms of tightness or pain.

Once the swelling has been reduced and the pain is diminished, you want to ease the compression and increase the circulation of blood to continue healing the area. Lemongrass and Cypress in the Carpal Tunnel Soother blend help ease the compressions, while the other ingredients promote healing.

Carpal Tunnel Soother

8 drops Cypress

10 drops Lemongrass

10 drops Marjoram

5 drops Peppermint

Add all essential oils to 2 ounces of base lotion or 2 tablespoons of of carrier oil (any oil listed in the "Carrier Oils" chapter). Apply a small amount of the blend to the affected area and the areas immediately above and below the affected area. Apply the blend 4 to 6 times a day for at least two weeks until the pain subsides.

If the pain does not subside after two weeks, continue to apply the blend 4 to 6 times daily for up to 6 weeks. Individual progress with carpal tunnel varies.

Muscle Aches and Pains

"Only two things are infinite, the universe and human stupidity, and I'm not sure about the former."

Albert Einstein

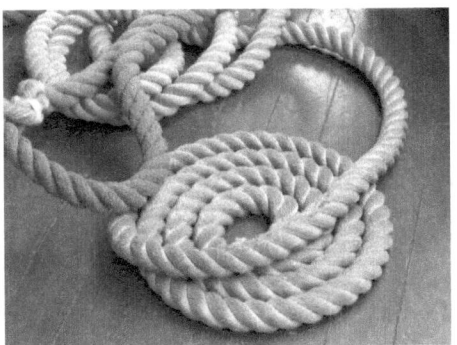

If you took a survey of every person who has ever had a muscle cramp or pain, you would probably find out that the cause of most of those injuries was something preventable. Einstein may call that human stupidity, and I'm sure at times we've called it that as well (or something worse). Nevertheless, if you are going to participate in sports of any kind, garden, or shop until you drop, you are going to get a muscle cramp or pain.

Muscle cramps are involuntary and often painful contractions of the muscles which produce a hard, bulging muscle. Some of the causes of muscle cramps are muscle fatigue, heavy exercise, dehydration, pregnancy, some medications, and physical overindulgence.

The best thing for you to do when you get a cramp is relax and slowly and gently stretch the affected muscle. If you do not get relief, consider contacting your physician. You should also call your doctor if you have severe, prolonged, or recurring muscle spasms or cramps that are unexplained or aren't relieved by simple stretching.

Muscle pain is discomfort involving any muscle. It is often caused by overuse, over exercising, or physically demanding work. In these situations, the muscle pain involves specific muscles or muscle groups and the cause of the muscle pain is fairly obvious. Keep in mind that stress can also cause muscle pain.

Rest is probably the most important aspect of healing. Apply ice for the first 24 hours, then switch to heat. Many physicians and physical therapists suggest that after 24 hours, you alternate 15 minutes of ice with 15 minutes of heat for up to three days. When the pain has eased to the point that you can tolerate it, try gentle stretching exercises and a gentle massage. To prevent more muscle pain, exercise on a regular basis. Start slowly and move from a subtle to more vigorous exercise routine. Walking and swimming are excellent exercise activities that provide muscle tone and good cardiovascular health.

For sore, strained muscles you can use muscle rub or liniment that has cayenne as an ingredient. You can buy the liniment over the counter or make your own: 1 tablespoon Cayenne in ½ cup hot vinegar, cool to a comfortable temperature. Mix with Olive oil and rub into muscles.

You should contact your doctor if the muscle pain persists beyond 3 days (that is if you rested and took care of it during those three days). Also call if you have a fever, rash, or swelling and bruising at the site of the muscle pain.

Essential Oil Blends

The following essential oils have good pain-relieving properties and promote healing: Chamomile (both German and Roman), Clary Sage, Clove, Eucalyptus, Ginger, Nutmeg, Black Pepper, Peppermint, Rosemary, and Thyme.

To draw out the pain, use Basil, Lemongrass, Marjoram, Nutmeg, Sage, and Spruce.

If the muscle is cramping, these essential oils can be helpful: Black Pepper, Cypress, Grapefruit, Lavender, Lemon, Marjoram, Pine, Rosemary, and Thyme. Refer to the "Essential Oil Chart" for contraindications, warnings, or cautions about using essential oils.

When you first injure your muscle, the Muscle Pain Relief blend is great for reducing the pain. However, keep in mind that pain reminds you not to overdo or shorten the healing process, so use this blend just enough to relieve the significant pain.

I've been called a "pain in the butt", however there was a softball season in which I actually experienced pain in my butt. I didn't realize that pitching 200 softballs to 12 girls during an evening practice had anything to do with my butt, until the next day, when just moving was painful.

To treat bruises, muscle aches, or sprains anywhere on your body, apply the essential oil blends in a straight upward motion; see the "Aches & Pains" section for details.

Muscle Pain Relief

10 drops Chamomile

8 drops Clove

8 drops Cypress

10 drops Lavender

> Mix all the oils together in a dark glass container. For the first 48 hours, apply a cold compress to the affected area as often as possible, up to 3 times per hour. Place 3 drops of the blend onto the cold wet cloth prior to each application. Keep the compress on the affected area until the cloth reaches room temperature.
>
> After 48 hours, add the remainder of the essential oils to 2 ounces of base lotion or 2 tablespoons carrier oil (any oil listed in the "Carrier Oils" chapter). Apply a small amount of the blend to the area of injury and the areas immediately above and below the site of injury. Apply the blend 4 to 6 times a day for the first 5 – 7 days until the pain subsides.

When the pain has eased, you may want to switch to the Muscle Pain Soother blend, because Eucalyptus promotes the health of red and white blood cells, which facilitates healing. This blend also contains pain-relieving oils.

Muscle Pain Soother

10 drops Eucalyptus

10 drops Marjoram

10 drops Spruce

> Add all the oils to 2 ounces of base lotion or 2 tablespoons carrier oil (any oil listed in the "Carrier Oils" chapter). Apply a small amount of the blend to the area of injury and the areas immediately above and below the site of injury. Apply the blend 4 to 6 times a day for the first 5 – 7 days until the pain subsides.

Muscle Cramps require immediate attention. To ease the pain and relax the cramp, use the Muscle Cramp Relief blend.

When one of my players came up to me complaining about a cramp in her calf muscle, I asked her what she did. "I was trying to see how many times I could bounce up and down on one leg," was her teary response. While the Cramp Relief blend did not necessarily help her thought process, I know it helped her muscle.

Muscle Cramp Relief

10 drops Clary Sage

8 drops Cypress

10 drops Marjoram

5 drops Rosemary

> Mix all essential oils in 2 tablespoons olive oil. Keep at room temperature, or slightly warmer. Before engaging in the activity that causes a muscle cramp (which can be anything from exercising to sleeping), apply the blend to the area most susceptible to cramping. If you already have the cramp, stretch the muscles surrounding the cramped area gently while applying the blend in an upward motion below, through, and above the cramped area.

To promote good muscle tone and avoid cramping, use the Muscle Cramp Prevention blend before and after you exercise.

Muscle Cramp Prevention

12 drops Lavender

12 drops Lemon

9 drops Peppermint

9 drops Rosemary

> Mix all essential oils in 2 tablespoons olive oil. Keep at room temperature, or slightly warmer. Before engaging in the activity that causes a muscle cramp (which can be anything from exercising to sleeping), apply the blend to the area most susceptible to cramping. If you already have the cramp, stretch the muscles surrounding the cramped area gently while applying the blend in an upward motion below, through, and above the cramped area.

Muscle Strain lets you know that you have overdone it, but you have not yet caused significant damage. However, the pain feels significant, and either of these Muscle Strain Relief blends can help.

Muscle Strain Relief 1

10 drops Chamomile

5 drops Clove

10 drops Ginger

5 drops Nutmeg

Mix all the oils together in a dark glass container. For the first 48 hours, apply a cold compress to the affected area as often as possible, up to 3 times per hour. Place 3 drops of the blend onto the cold wet cloth prior to each application. Keep the compress on the affected area until the cloth reaches room temperature.

After 48 hours, add the remainder of the essential oils to 2 ounces of base lotion or 2 tablespoons carrier oil (any oil listed in the "Carrier Oils" chapter). Apply a small amount of the blend to the area of injury and the areas immediately above and below the site of injury. Apply the blend 4 to 6 times a day for the first 5 – 7 days until the pain subsides.

Muscle Strain Relief 2

5 drops Black Pepper

8 drops Cypress

10 drops Lavender

10 drops Marjoram

> Mix all the oils together in a dark glass container. For the first 48 hours, apply a cold compress to the affected area as often as possible, up to 3 times per hour. Place 3 drops of the blend onto the cold wet cloth prior to each application. Keep the compress on the affected area until the cloth reaches room temperature.
>
> After 48 hours, add the remainder of the essential oils to 2 ounces of base lotion or 2 tablespoons carrier oil (any oil listed in the "Carrier Oils" chapter). Apply a small amount of the blend to the area of injury and the areas immediately above and below the site of injury. Apply the blend 4 to 6 times a day for the first 5 – 7 days until the pain subsides.

Use the Muscle Strain Support blend after your muscles are healed to continue to provide support to the large muscles.

Muscle Strain Support

10 drops Eucalyptus

10 drops Peppermint

10 drops Rosemary

> Mix all oils together. Use in any of these ways:

> Put 10 drops in 2 tablespoons of carrier oil and massage the affected area. The ideal time to do this is after a warm bath and before bedtime.

> Put 8 drops in a bath. Relax your cares away while you deep soak the strain from your muscles.

Sore muscles often occur because you are using a muscle group that you don't use often. When this happens, use the Sore Muscles Relief blend to provide pain relief and to promote healing.

Sore Muscles Relief

10 drops Chamomile

10 drops Clary Sage

10 drops Lavender

5 drops Rosemary

> Mix all the oils together in a dark glass container. For the first 48 hours, apply a cold compress to the affected area as often as possible, up to 3 times per hour. Place 3 drops of the blend onto the cold wet cloth prior to each application. Keep the compress on the affected area until the cloth reaches room temperature.

> After 48 hours, add the remainder of the essential oils to 2 ounces of base lotion or 2 tablespoons carrier oil (any oil listed in the "Carrier Oils" chapter). Apply a small amount of the blend to the area of injury and the areas immediately above and below the site of injury. Apply the blend 4 to 6 times a day for the first 5 – 7 days until the pain subsides.

To promote good muscle tone and avoid injury, use the Sore Muscle Support blend before and after you exercise.

Sore Muscle Support

10 drops Juniper

10 drops Lavender

10 drops Marjoram

5 drops Rosemary

> Mix all essential oils in 2 tablespoons olive oil. Keep at room temperature, or slightly warmer. Before engaging in the activity that causes sore muscles, apply the blend to the muscle group in an upward motion below, through, and above the area.

Neck Pain

*"The secret of success is learning how to use pain and pleasure
instead of having pain and pleasure use you. If you do that, you're
in control of your life. If you don't, life controls you."*

Anthony Robbins

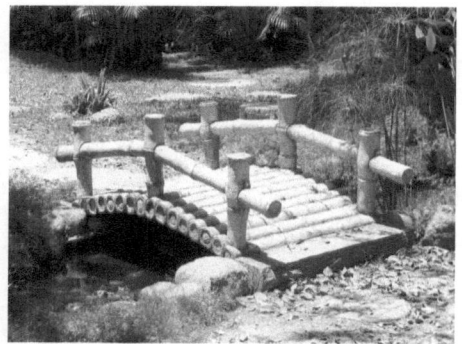

You've got to believe that Anthony Robbins has suffered both pain
and pleasure during his successful journey into entrepreneurship.
And, at his height, his neck has probably suffered a great deal
through constantly tilting downwards to look at people or upwards
in fulfillment of his dreams.

There are many causes of neck pain. If you wake with neck pain, you might be sleeping in an improper manner. Accidents can cause neck pain even though you may also experience discomfort in your arms and back. Repetitive activity, such as working on a computer all day, may also cause neck pain. One of the best things you can do is determine the source of your neck pain.

Once you identify the cause, you can change your behavior to correct it. Neck pain, however, is slow to improve and may take several weeks to go away, so stick with a relief strategy as well as a prevention plan. Warm compresses, gentle massage, and rest are all helpful in getting relief from your neck pain.

If you experience fever, headache, numbness, or tingling in the arm, call your doctor immediately. If the pain lasts for more than a couple of weeks or you start getting swollen glands, call your doctor.

Essential Oil Blends

Neck pain reacts very well to essential oils such as Black Pepper, Chamomile, Clove, Eucalyptus, Ginger, Lavender, Marjoram, Peppermint, Rosemary, and Thyme. Refer to the "Essential Oil Chart" for any contraindications, warnings, or cautions about using essential oils.

When you first sprain your neck or any other muscle/joint, the Neck Pain Relief blend is great for reducing the pain. However, keep in mind that pain reminds you not to overdo or shorten the healing process, so use this blend just enough to relieve the significant pain.

To treat bruises, muscle aches, or sprains anywhere on your body, apply the essential oil blends in a straight upward motion; see the "Aches & Pains" section for details.

When I injured my neck in an auto accident, the Neck Pain Relief blend worked so well that my chiropractor now uses it in his practice.

Neck Pain Relief

10 drops Lavender

10 drops Marjoram

5 drops Peppermint

8 drops Spruce

> Mix all the oils together in a dark glass container. For the first 48 hours, apply a cold compress to the affected area as often as possible, up to 3 times per hour. Place 3 drops of the blend onto the cold wet cloth prior to each application. Keep the compress on the affected area until the cloth reaches room temperature.

> After 48 hours, add the remainder of the essential oils to 2 ounces of base lotion or 2 tablespoons carrier oil (any oil listed in the "Carrier Oils" chapter). Apply a small amount of the blend to the area of injury and the areas immediately above and below the site of injury. Apply the blend 4 to 6 times a day for the first 5 – 7 days until the pain subsides.

When the pain has eased, you may want to switch to the Neck Pain Soother blend because it also contains oils that have the ability to draw deep-seated pain out. *This blend is very effective for people with chronic neck pain due to sitting at a computer all day long and for those who hold stress in their neck area.*

Neck Pain Soother

5 drops Black Pepper

10 drops Ginger

10 drops Lavender

5 drops Peppermint

Add all the oils to 2 ounces of base lotion or 2 tablespoons carrier oil (any oil listed in the "Carrier Oils" chapter). Apply a small amount of the blend to the area of injury and the areas immediately above and below the site of injury. Apply the blend 4 to 6 times a day for the first 5 – 7 days until the pain subsides.

Pain Relief

"I do not feel obliged to believe that the same God who has endowed us with sense, reason, and intellect has intended us to forgo their use."

Galileo Galilei

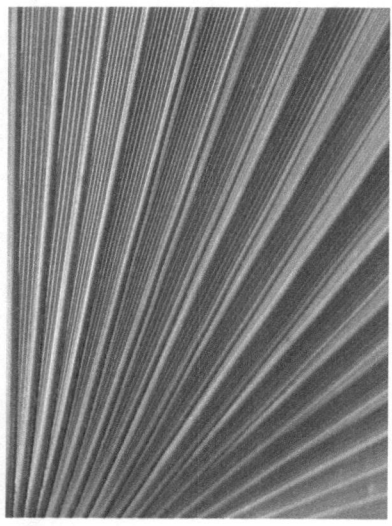

And yet, that's exactly how we may feel when we do something that causes pain. Of course, not every pain is caused because we have forgotten to use our sense, reason, and intellect; but lack of judgment and good sense is at the root of many injuries.

Pain serves as an alert to potential or actual damage to the body. The definition for damage is quite broad; pain can arise from injury as well as disease. Once the brain has received and processed the pain message and coordinated an appropriate response, pain has served its purpose. The body uses natural painkillers, called endorphins, to derail further pain messages.

Pain is generally divided into two categories: acute and chronic. Acute pain is associated with injury, headaches, disease, and other conditions. It usually goes away once the condition that precipitated it is resolved. The time limit used to define chronic pain typically ranges from three to six months, although some healthcare professionals prefer a more flexible definition and consider chronic pain any pain that lasts beyond a normal healing time.

Pain can have a negative impact on a person's mental health and impede recovery from illness or injury. Unrelieved pain can become a syndrome in its own right and cause a downward spiral in a person's health and outlook. Managing pain properly facilitates recovery, prevents additional health complications, and improves an individual's quality of life.

To control chronic pain, try relaxation techniques, such as yoga and meditation. Participating in normal activities and exercising can also help control pain levels by producing endorphins.

Consult your physician if you cannot identify the cause of the pain, the pain seems to intensify, or if you have other symptoms such as nausea, fever, or rash.

Essential Oil Blends

Pain responds well to essential oils including Chamomile, Clove, Cypress, Eucalyptus, Ginger, Lavender, Marjoram, Nutmeg, Black Pepper, Peppermint, Rosemary, Thyme, and Vetiver. Refer to the "Essential Oil Chart" for contraindications, warnings, or cautions about using essential oils.

When you first experience pain, the Pain Relief blend is great for reducing the pain. However, keep in mind that pain reminds you not to overdo or shorten the healing process, so use this blend just enough to relieve the significant pain.

Nobody wants to experience pain of any kind, but pain can be viewed as a positive message from your body, because it warns you that you are doing something that is damaging, and needs to be addressed. Don't think that because you are in pain, you are a wimp (like my brothers so ruthlessly teased me); realize that pain may be telling you something important.

To treat bruises, muscle aches, or sprains anywhere on your body, apply the essential oil blends in a straight upward motion; see the "Aches & Pains" section for details.

Pain Relief

5 drops Chamomile

5 drops Lavender

5 drops Lemon

5 drops Peppermint

10 drops Rosemary

> Mix all oils together. Add the essential oils to 2 tablespoons olive oil. Gently massage the blend into painful muscles.

When the pain has eased, you may want to switch to the Pain Soother blend because it also contains oils that can draw deep-seated pain out.

Pain Soother

10 drops Chamomile

5 drops Clove

8 drops Cypress

8 drops Ginger

8 drops Nutmeg

Add all the to 2 ounces of base lotion or 2 tablespoons carrier oil (any oil listed in the "Carrier Oils" chapter). Apply a small amount of the blend to the area of injury and the areas immediately above and below the site of injury. Apply the blend 4 to 6 times a day for the first 5 – 7 days until the pain subsides.

You may want to continue to use the blend once daily simply to avoid the recurrence of pain.

Tendonitis

"Pain is no evil unless it conquers us."

George Eliot

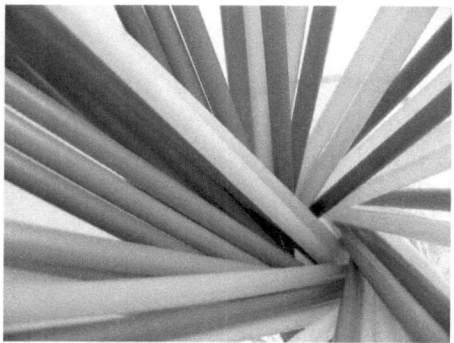

And conquer us it does — at times. For people who have triggered damage to their tendons because of recreational activities such as tennis, golf, or bowling, giving up those activities for a period of time to recover isn't that awful. However, for a person whose livelihood depends upon the constant strain on a tendon, such as my friend who is a banquet waitress and another friend who owns a horse farm and must muck out stalls daily, tendonitis can impact your income. Fortunately, essential oils can help relieve the pain and support the tendons to let you keep working without pain.

Frequently called tennis elbow, tendonitis can result from sudden stretching or repeated overuse of the connection between the tendon and its bone or muscle. The body tries to heal by initiating inflammation to increase the blood supply and bring nutrients to the damaged tissues. The result is congestion, which causes swelling, tenderness, pain, heat, and redness if the inflammation is close to the skin.

Tendonitis usually happens to people in middle or old age because it is often the result of overuse over a long period of time. The common sites of tendonitis are the hand, elbow, upper arm, shoulder, and the Achilles tendon.

Rest, ice, compression, and elevation (RICE) will treat the acute condition. Generally, tendonitis will heal if you stop the provoking activity. If given enough time, tendons will strengthen to meet the demands placed on them.

Consult your physician if the pain seems to intensify or if you are experiencing any other symptoms such as nausea, fever, or rash.

Essential Oil Blends

Essential oils that can help promote nerve health and circulation are: Basil, Cypress, Eucalyptus, Ginger, Lavender, Lemongrass, Marjoram, Peppermint, and Rosemary. Refer to the "Essential Oil Chart" for contraindications, warnings, or cautions about using essential oils.

The first symptoms of tendonitis are tightness in the muscles followed by tingling in the arm and throbbing pain. To reduce the swelling and relieve the pain, use one of the Tendonitis Relief blends.

To treat bruises, muscle aches, or sprains anywhere on your body, apply the essential oil blends in a straight upward motion; see the "Aches & Pains" section for details.

When I coached my daughter's softball team, I would pitch about 200 balls during every practice. I really thought my arm grew an inch after every practice. I also thought that alternating between ice and heat would just become a regular part of the softball season. When I added the Tendonitis Relief blends to the cold and hot compresses, I experienced more significant relief.

Tendonitis Relief 1

8 drops Ginger

10 drops Lavender

10 drops Peppermint

10 drops Rosemary

> Mix all the oils together in a dark glass container. For the first 48 hours, apply a cold compress to the affected area as often as possible, up to 3 times per hour. Place 3 drops of the blend on the cold wet cloth prior to each application. Keep the compress on the affected area until the cloth reaches room temperature.
>
> After 48 hours, add the remainder of the essential oils to 2 ounces of base lotion or 2 tablespoons carrier oil (any oil listed in the "Carrier Oils" chapter). Apply a small amount of the blend to the area of injury and the areas immediately above and below the site of injury. Apply the blend 4 to 6 times a day for the first 5 – 7 days until the pain subsides.

Tendonitis Relief 2

6 drops Cypress

8 drops Eucalyptus

8 drops Peppermint

8 drops Rosemary

> Mix all the oils together in a dark glass container. For the first 48 hours, apply a cold compress to the affected area as often as possible, up to 3 times per hour. Place 3 drops of the blend on the cold wet cloth prior to each application. Keep the compress on the affected area until the cloth reaches room temperature.
>
> After 48 hours, add the remainder of the essential oils to 2 ounces of base lotion or 2 tablespoons carrier oil (any oil listed in the "Carrier Oils" chapter). Apply a small amount of the blend to the area of injury and the areas immediately above and below the site of injury. Apply the blend 4 to 6 times a day for the first 5 – 7 days until the pain subsides.

Once the swelling has been reduced and the pain is diminished, you want to draw out any remaining congestion and increase the circulation of blood to continue healing the area. Lemongrass and Ginger in the Tendonitis Soother blend helps draw out congestion, while the other ingredients promote healing.

Tendonitis Soother

12 drops Ginger

8 drops Lemongrass

10 drops Marjoram

> Add all the oils to 2 ounces of base lotion or 2 tablespoons carrier oil (any oil listed in the "Carrier Oils" chapter). Apply a small amount of the blend to the area of injury and the areas immediately above and below the site of injury. Apply the blend 4 to 6 times a day for the first 5 – 7 days until you are comfortable.

All About Skin

What's the best way to use essential oils for skin care?

One of the best methods of enjoying essential oils is to place the essential oils into a bath. First, the oils would be able to penetrate all of your skin. Second, you would also get benefit from the smell of the essential oils as the warm water diffuses them. Finally, you get benefit from the fact that you took time to give yourself some tender loving care.

While you can put essential oils directly into a bath, let me give you a recipe for a basic bath salt. You can start with one cup of Epsom salts and add 6 – 12 drops of essential oils. Then, use as little as a quarter cup of the bath salts or overindulge and use the entire cup in your next bath. The beauty of this simple recipe is twofold; first, you are using natural ingredients, and second, it only costs you pennies to enjoy so many tremendous advantages.

For a nourishing and moisturizing bath salt, mix 1 cup of powdered milk, ¼ cup baking soda, and ¼ cup Epsom salts; then add 12 – 18 drops of essential oils.

The remainder of this section deals with:

- Acne
- Dermatitis
- Dry Skin
- Eczema
- Rash
- Scar Tissue
- Shaving and Razor Burn
- Wrinkles

Acne

"Retirement at sixty-five is ridiculous. When I was sixty-five I still had pimples."

George Burns

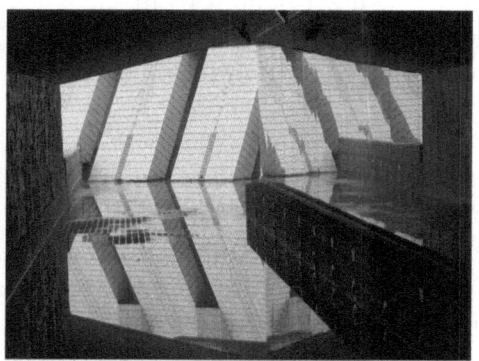

Unbelievable — we can still get acne when we are sixty-five. Acne assumes different forms and people react differently towards it. For some, there is little inflammation, while others have boulders the size of an orange (all right maybe not quite so large, but it feels that way). Some people get acne only when their hormones are fluctuating and others have it all the time (all right, not from birth, but soon after it seems). Acne always seems to pop up (get it?) at the worst possible moment — before a job interview, the day of the prom — you know how it is.

Regardless of your age or what has influenced your body to react, acne begins the same way — an enlarged hair follicle plugged with oil causes the surrounding skin to become inflamed.

The research is split on what causes acne, but some of the culprits are allergies, stress, hormones, perspiration, the use of certain drugs; junk foods, saturated fats, hydrogenated fats, animal products, nutritional deficiencies, exposure to industrial pollutants, the use of cosmetics, and over-washing or repeated rubbing of the skin.

When you look at the statistics, just about everyone gets acne at some point in their life. The secret to controlling acne is prevention (easier said than done), but you can control the visible signs of acne.

You will find your breakouts lessen if you clean up other aspects of your life. Try these:

- Drink plenty of water daily.

- Take a multiple vitamin and check with your doctor about other vitamins, minerals, or supplements that might be useful.

- Eat fruits and vegetables. Try to avoid sugar, white flour, and deep fried foods.

- Get your circulation working with aerobic exercise.

- Wash your face thoroughly, but not roughly. Use a gentle soap — don't use a deodorant soap on your face.

Essential Oil Blends

The best essential oils for acne are Chamomile, Clary Sage, Eucalyptus, Geranium, Juniper, Lavender, Lemon, Peppermint, Rosemary, and Tea Tree. Refer to the "Essential Oil Chart" for contraindications, warnings, or cautions about using essential oils.

The Blemish Blocker and Acne Eraser blends are potent. Apply the oils directly on the acne. Both of these blends work well on one or two pimples. Don't use them over large areas of skin because each blend is very drying.

The Blemish Blocker recipe is from my first aromatherapy book. So many people have had such terrific results that I wanted to be sure to share the recipe with you.

Blemish Blocker

10 drops Lavender

10 drops Lemon

10 drops Tea Tree

> Mix all the oils together in a dark glass container. Use a cotton ball or Q-tip to apply tiny amounts to spots on your skin. Let air dry, then use your facial moisturizer.

> Blemish Blocker may sting when you apply it. Don't use it too often, because it is also very drying. The acne should diminish within 5 – 7 days.

Keep in mind to use the Acne Eraser blend only on sporadic pimples. The ingredients help extract the blocked skin oils and also reduce inflammation.

Acne Eraser

10 drops Fennel

10 drops Lavender

10 drops Lemon

> Mix all the oils together in a dark glass container. Use a cotton ball or Q-tip to apply tiny amounts to spots on your skin. Let air dry, then use your facial moisturizer.
>
> Acne Eraser may sting when you apply it. Don't use it too often, because it is also very drying. The acne should diminish within 5 – 7 days.

The following blend is good for treating acne on large areas such as chest and back. You can also use it on your face as a toner.

My daughter is just beginning to experience acne and changes in the oiliness of her facial skin. She is not a happy camper. We use the Acne Relief Spray on her face as a daily toner. In addition, I made a light natural face moisturizer – both these products seem to take care of things. It is important to remember that your skin seeks balance; too much dryness or oiliness is going to cause skin eruptions of some sort. Therefore, I recommend both a toner and a moisturizer.

Acne Relief Spray

4 drops Chamomile

6 drops Clary Sage

4 drops Geranium

10 drops Lavender

2 drops Tea Tree

Add all of the essential oils, 2 ounces of cider vinegar, and 2 ounces of witch hazel to 8 ounces of water. Place contents into a spray bottle and shake well.

Spritz (3 – 5 squirts) the affected area lightly at least twice a day for 7 to 10 days. You should notice improvement during that period of time. Continue to use the blend twice daily until acne diminishes. You can use the blend up to four times daily. Be sure to close your eyes when you spray your face.

Dermatitis

"It is the part of a good shepherd to shear his flock, not to skin it."

Latin proverb

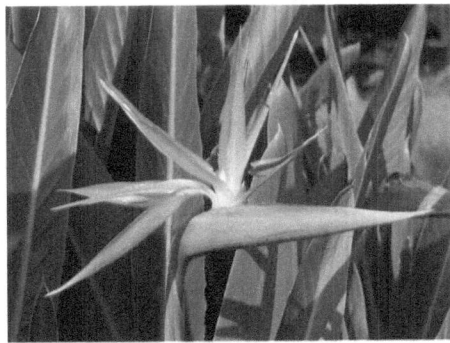

You feel like you are being skinned alive when the itchiness and inflammation of dermatitis is at its worst.

Many skin disorders, such as dermatitis, eczema, and psoriasis, are often difficult to diagnose and therefore difficult to treat. Symptoms of dermatitis include inflammation, redness, itchiness, and swelling on various parts of the body. The most common sites are the scalp, sides of the nose, eyebrows, eyelids, skin behind the ears, and the middle of the chest. However, the navel (belly button) and skin folds under the arms, breasts, groin, and buttocks may also be involved.

To make matters worse, the cause of most skin disorders is unknown, and while many are easily treated, the disorder frequently reoccurs. Dermatitis has been defined as "an inflammatory condition of the skin caused by outside agents." The outside agents that cause dermatitis may be cleaning products, solvents, or metals (as in jewelry).

At the onset of dermatitis, take a few minutes and review the past few days. What did you eat? What did you use to wash your clothing and bed sheets? Did you have any unusual stressors going on? Did you try a new cologne or perfume? Think about this in as much detail as possible and jot down some notes. You might just find the culprit and stay healthy by avoiding it.

It seems that no age group is free of dermatitis as it can affect infants (cradle cap), middle-aged people, and the elderly, and appears to be most common in people with oily skin or hair.

Gentle care of the affected area is the best treatment for dermatitis, which has a high tendency to recur. Mild shampoos, gentle moisturizing treatments, and low strength medical products are effective and reduce the risk of side effects. Of course, when in doubt, consult your dermatologist or physician. Vitamin C is helpful in dealing with the inflammation present with dermatitis.

Essential Oil Blends

The best essential oils for healing skin and counteracting the inflammation of dermatitis are Carrot, Cedar, Chamomile, Clary Sage, Frankincense, Geranium, Juniper, Lavender, Palmarosa, Patchouli, Peppermint, Orange, Rosemary, Rosewood, Sage, Sandalwood, Tea Tree, and Thyme. Refer to the "Essential Oil

Chart" for contraindications, warnings, or cautions about using essential oils.

This Daytime Dermatitis Relief blend is healing and cooling. However, Peppermint has stimulant properties so you may not want to use this blend just before bedtime.

Daytime Dermatitis Relief

10 drops Chamomile

10 drops Geranium

20 drops Lavender

4 drops Peppermint

> Mix all the oils together in a dark glass container.
>
> Add 8 – 12 drops of the blended oils to your bath. If you have time only for a shower, put 5 – 7 drops on your wet cloth and smooth over your body after washing.
>
> Add 32 drops of the essential oils to 2 ounces of base lotion or 2 tablespoons of carrier oil (any oil listed in the "Carrier Oils" chapter). Apply a small amount of the blend to the affected area 4 to 6 times a day until the dermatitis subsides. You can expect relief within 7 - 10 days.

The Evening Dermatitis Relief blend also contains some wonderful essential oils to heal your skin. In addition, the Chamomile, Lavender, and Geranium also have very calming properties that will help you relax. This is a blend you should use at the end of your day.

Evening Dermatitis Relief

12 drops Chamomile

8 drops Geranium

15 drops Lavender

15 drops Patchouli

Mix all the oils together in a dark glass container.

Add 8 – 12 drops of the blended oils to your bath. If you have time only for a shower, put 5 – 7 drops on your wet cloth and smooth over your body after washing.

Add 32 drops of the essential oils to 2 ounces of base lotion or 2 tablespoons of carrier oil (any oil listed in the "Carrier Oils" chapter). Apply a small amount of the blend to the affected area 4 to 6 times a day until the dermatitis subsides. You can expect relief within 7 - 10 days.

Often when your skin is cracked and irritated by dermatitis, you are extra susceptible to germs and infections. The Dermatitis Treatment blend provides strong antibiotic relief with Tea Tree, Lavender, and Cedarwood, as well as anti-inflammatory relief with Chamomile.

Dermatitis Treatment

14 drops Cedarwood

16 drops Chamomile

16 drops Lavender

14 drops Tea Tree

Mix all the oils together in a dark glass container.

Add 8 – 12 drops of the blended oils to your bath. If you have time only for a shower, put 5 – 7 drops on your wet cloth and smooth over your body after washing.

Add 32 drops of the essential oils to 2 ounces of base lotion or 2 tablespoons of carrier oil (any oil listed in the "Carrier Oils" chapter). Apply a small amount of the blend to the affected area 4 to 6 times a day until the dermatitis subsides. You can expect relief within 7 - 10 days.

Dry Skin

"In the dry desert of a thousand lines"

Alexander Pope

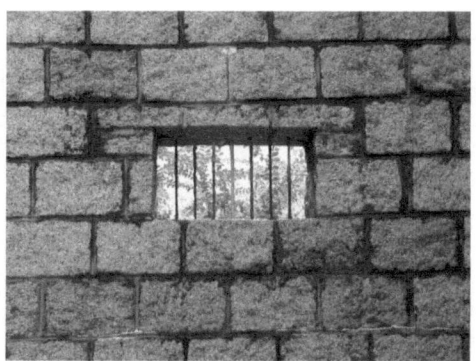

Last winter was a long, snow-filled season. Hank, who plows snow in New England, did so often. He plowed, shoveled, and put chains on the tires of his truck, all without wearing gloves. Several weeks into winter Hank had dry skin that cracked, itched, and burned. His sister, Mary, owns a daycare center in Georgia. Between washing her hands constantly and cleaning the facility to keep it as antiseptic and disinfected as possible, she also suffered with raw, chapped skin.

Each day, your actions are potentially dangerous to your skin: too much time in the sun, too much time in water, a paper cut. Your inaction is also potentially dangerous to your skin: you forget sunscreen, you don't wear gloves to wash dishes, and you don't wear moisturizer. To have whole, comfortable, and beautiful skin you have responsibilities. You need to cure any problems you are presently having with your skin. You need to avoid potentially damaging things for your skin. You need to pamper your skin.

As you age, your skin loses elasticity and becomes thinner. This makes it easier to injure your skin. And, often the lower quality of your nutrition makes it harder for your skin to heal. Anyone who has experienced those little cracks that appear on the tips of fingers that stretch apart in chapped hands knows how long it takes for your skin to literally come together again.

So what can you do? For many people dry skin is preventable. If you are careful not to expose yourself to too much wind, cold, or sun; if you avoid contact with harsh synthetic soaps and chemicals, and if you wear clothes that let your skin breathe; then you may not get dry skin very often. Other time-tested remedies include Bag Balm and Udder Cream (available at farm or feed stores) and Crisco.

You can help from the inside, too. Your diet can affect your skin's tendency to dry out. If your diet is not high enough in fat you will experience more problems with dry skin. Keep your nutrition balanced. Some fat is good for you. Eating vitamin A-rich foods such as carrots, tomatoes, and leafy vegetables can help repair skin. Also foods rich in vitamin B5, such as whole grains, legumes, wheat germ, and nutritional yeast, can promote essential fatty acids, which help moisturize the skin. Drinking lots of water keeps your skin hydrated. Exercise also benefits the skin as it boosts circulation and encourages blood flow.

Essential Oil Blends

The best essential oils for your skin are Carrot, Chamomile, Clary Sage, Geranium, Lavender, Patchouli, Rosewood, and Sandalwood. *There are more expensive essential oils that you can use to improve your skin. However, try these less expensive oils first; save the money to do something fun!* Refer to the "Essential Oil Chart" for contraindications, warnings, or cautions about using essential oils.

You will find the Extra Dry Skin Relief blend soothing and healing. *The Extra Dry Skin Relief is one of my most popular blends because it works so well on people of all ages. It also works quite effectively on freshly shaved areas and to treat sunburn.*

Extra Dry Skin Relief

10 drops Carrot

20 drops Chamomile

20 drops Geranium

16 drops Lavender

> Mix all the oils together in a dark glass container.
>
> For bathing: Add 8 – 12 drops of the blended oils into your bath. If you prefer a shower, put 5 – 7 drops on a wet facecloth cloth and smooth over your body after you rinse. You won't need to wash off the essential oils.
>
> For a lotion: Add 32 drops of the essential oils to 2 ounces of base lotion or 2 tablespoons of a carrier oil (any oil listed in the "Carrier Oils" chapter). Apply a small amount of the blend to your dry skin 4 to 6 times a day until the dry skin subsides. You can expect relief within 3 – 5 days.

Use the Skin Soother blend when you have time to allow the carrier oil to be absorbed by your skin. You will find it well worth the extra minutes. Combine the relaxing and soothing benefits of a massage with a blend that makes you feel silky and spoiled; that sounds right to me.

Skin Soother

2 drop Cedarwood

6 drops Clary Sage

2 drop Geranium

2 drop Lavender

6 drops Rosemary

> Mix the essential oils together in 2 tablespoons of olive oil. Massage (or have your partner massage) your entire body with this relaxing blend. Don't forget those extra dry areas like elbows, knees, and ankles. Use this once a day. You can expect relief within 3 – 5 days.

For nighttime, you can use the Dry Skin Night Time Moisturizer. Besides being good for your skin, it has a wonderful scent and is very relaxing.

Dry Skin Night Time Moisturizer

7 drops Geranium

3 drops Rosewood

10 drops Sandalwood

5 drops Ylang Ylang

> Combine the essential oils with 2 ounces carrier oils. Use this as a moisturizer after cleansing in the evening. Most of the carrier oils will absorb quickly. However, if this feels too greasy for you, you can use your favorite non-scented lotion as the carrier.

If you can't find someone to give you a massage, pamper yourself with the Dry Skin After Bath Oil blend.

Dry Skin After Bath Oil

12 drops Carrot

12 drops Chamomile

6 drops Geranium

6 drops Myrrh

6 drops Patchouli

18 drops Rosewood

> Combine the essential oils with 2 ounces carrier oil (use Sweet Almond, Apricot, Avocado, or Olive) and use as a body moisturizer immediately after your bath or shower when your skin is still somewhat moist.

The Chapped Hands Cure blend is really a first aid treatment. Some of the oils are a bit more expensive, but this blend works extremely well for badly chapped hands.

Chapped Hands Cure

2 drops Frankincense

2 drops Patchouli

3 drops Rosewood

3 drops Sandalwood

> Mix the essential oils in 2 ounces of cocoa butter. Use frequently on your chapped hands. This will heal even those little cracks that begin to pull apart.

> A great way to help this blend work is to apply the blend, wrap plastic wrap around your hands and put socks over them. Wear this to bed. It may not be attractive, but in the morning you will notice an immense difference in the condition of your hands.

Eczema

"Beauty is only skin deep, but ugly goes clear to the bone."

Parker's Law

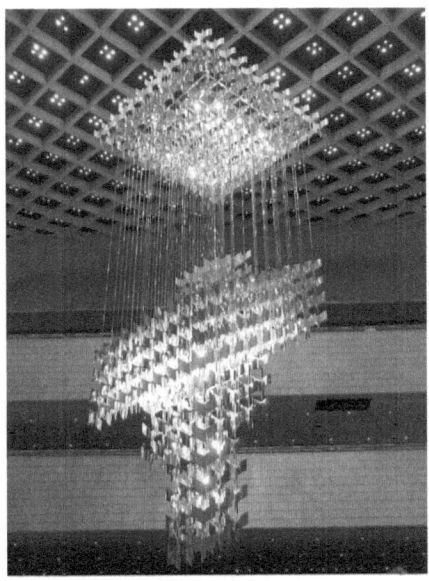

You might feel as if your eczema is digging so deeply into your skin that it is going clear to the bone. It's uncomfortable both physically and mentally. You have this skin condition that never lets you forget it.

Eczema is a chronic (long-lasting) non-contagious disease that causes the skin behind the ears, on the cheeks, arms, and legs to become extremely itchy and inflamed. This causes redness, swelling, cracking, weeping, crusting, and scaling. To make matters worse, scratching the area (a natural response) worsens the skin inflammation.

While eczema most often affects infants and young children, it can appear at any age. Men and women suffer equally from this skin disease. There is no known cause, but scientists do believe that hereditary and environmental factors may contribute to eczema. Unfortunately, there is no test to diagnose eczema and no single symptom or feature used to identify the disease. Also, for many who suffer from eczema, stress, soaps, detergents, perfumes, cosmetics, dust, and cigarette smoke worsen the condition.

Most eczema sufferers successfully treat the condition with proper skin care and lifestyle changes that can heal the skin and keep it healthy. When symptoms do occur try the following suggestions: lukewarm baths with non-soap cleansers, skin moisturizers, soft cotton fabrics, and by avoiding overheating. You can also get relief from the essential oil blends described here.

Essential Oil Blends

The best essential oils for healing skin and counteracting the inflammation of eczema are Cedarwood, Chamomile, Cypress, Lavender, Patchouli, Rosemary, Tea Tree, Thyme, and Yarrow. Refer to the "Essential Oil Chart" for contraindications, warnings, or cautions about using essential oils.

Even using the tender-yet-potent care of the essential oil blends in this section; you may find that your eczema symptoms appear to get worse before they get better. This is because as that bacteria is being expelled from your body, it is leaving fighting and screaming.

When you are treating Eczema, there is a fine balance that you must maintain to get the infection out of the body without damaging the skin further. In fact, if you choose to treat eczema through conventional medications, take Vitamin E and use natural skin moisturizing and soothing lotions. One of the great things about both of the following blends is that they mix strong anti-fungal, antibacterial, and antiseptic essential oils with skin moisturizing and soothing essential oils.

The Eczema Relief blend is power-packed to help draw out the bacteria and inflammation that is causing your skin to react.

Eczema Relief

20 drops Chamomile

10 drops Cypress

4 drops Tea Tree

10 drops Yarrow

> Mix all the oils together in a dark glass container. Use this blend in either of the following ways:
>
> Add 8 – 12 drops of the blended oils to your bath. If you have time only for a shower, put 5 – 7 drops on your wet cloth and smooth over your body after washing with a non soap cleanser.
>
> Add 32 drops of the essential oils to 2 ounces of base lotion or 2 tablespoons of carrier oil (any oil listed in the "Carrier Oils" chapter). Apply a small amount of the blend to the affected area 4 to 6 times a day until the eczema subsides. You can expect relief within 7 - 10 days.

The Eczema Soother blend is great for children 3 years and older. For children under 3 years of age, you can use this blend BUT replace the Thyme with Yarrow.

Eczema Soother

14 drops Chamomile

8 drops Geranium

8 drops Lavender

8 drops Patchouli

8 drops Thyme

Mix all the oils together in a dark glass container. Use this blend in either of the following ways:

Add 8 – 12 drops of the blended oils to your bath. If you have time only for a shower, put 5 – 7 drops on your wet cloth and smooth over body after washing.

Add 32 drops of the essential oils to 2 ounces of base lotion or 2 tablespoons of carrier oil (any oil listed in the "Carrier Oils" chapter). Apply a small amount of the blend to the affected area 4 to 6 times a day until the eczema subsides. You can expect relief within 7 - 10 days.

Rashes

"Take calculated risks. That is quite different from being rash."

George S. Patton

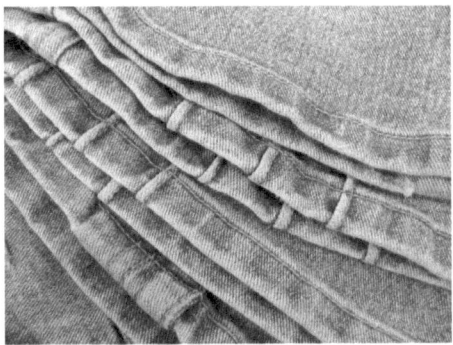

While the word "rash" can mean hasty, impulsive, and reckless as General Patton meant, rash also means a skin complaint, hives, pimples, itchiness, inflammation, and irritation. Before you act in a rash manner against your rash, learn a bit more.

Rash is a general term that describes a group of spots, an area of inflammation, or changes in the color or texture of the skin. Some rashes offer no discomfort at all. But, itching, tingling, burning, pain, or swelling may also accompany rashes. Some rashes appear over large areas of the body, while others show up in specific areas. Skin rashes may or may not be contagious. Some may be short-lived, while others are recurrent or chronic.

Diaper rash, chicken pox, athlete's foot, rosacea, shingles — it seems that we are susceptible to rashes our entire lives. The precise cause of most skin rashes is unknown, but the following are all associated with causing skin rashes: bacteria, viruses, fungi, insect bites, food allergies, abrasion, heat or sun exposure, chemical pollutants, medications, chemicals found in household cleaners, and cosmetics. Some things make you more susceptible to rashes, like stress, hormonal changes, genetic predisposition, and autoimmune problems.

See your family doctor or dermatologist if, in addition to the rash, you have a fever, swollen lymph nodes, infection, a bull's eye-shaped rash, headache, shortness of breath, sensitivity to light, a stiff neck, or achy joints.

The best way to treat a rash is avoidance – don't get a rash. Eat a healthy diet, exercise regularly, keep skin clean and moisturized, and protect skin from excesses, such as sun. If you do get a rash, the following hints will help:

- Use a mild soap, or just water, to clean the affected area.

- Use warm, not hot, water.

- Don't scrub your skin; be gentle.

- Dry your skin gently.

- Keep your skin moisturized.

- Wear natural fibers like cotton.

- Apply cool or lukewarm compresses to itchy or sore areas. Sprinkle the rash with baking soda.

- Avoid or minimize exposure to potential irritants, like harsh household cleaning products.

- Humidify the air in your home if you have dry skin, especially in the winter months.

Another familiar rash is diaper rash; see the "Diaper Rash" chapter for details.

Essential Oil Blends

The best essential oils for rashes are Carrot, Chamomile, Eucalyptus, Lavender, and Tea Tree. Refer to the "Essential Oil Chart" for contraindications, warnings, or cautions about using essential oils.

I think that a rash is one of the most obnoxious and uncomfortable things, so I try to pamper myself if and when I get one. In addition to using one of the essential oil recipes in this chapter, I take a tepid bath with baking soda, oatmeal, or Epsom salts. I like the fact that my entire body is being treated — you know how some of these rashes spread. I also like the candlelight and soft music I listen to in the bath. Remember to gently pat yourself dry after the bath and apply one of the oil-based blends here to moisturize your skin.

There are specific blends for diaper rash and cradle cap for our infants and toddlers. But if your child has a rash on other parts of their body, especially of an unknown origin, try the Children's Rash Treatment blend. The anti-fungal, germicidal, and antibacterial properties of the Tea Tree ensure that the area is clean and the Lavender and Bergamot help to heal the skin.

Children's Rash Treatment

16 drops Bergamot

20 drops Lavender

16 drops Tea Tree

Mix all the oils together in a dark glass container.

Put 22 drops of the blended oils in 8 ounces of water in a spray bottle. When you get a rash, spray the area with this blend, then let air dry.

Add 30 drops of the essential oils to 4 ounces of base lotion or 4 tablespoons of carrier oil (any oil listed in the "Carrier Oils" chapter). Apply a small amount of the blend to the affected area 4 to 6 times a day until the rash heals. You can expect relief within 1 - 3 days.

Some rashes cause itching. This causes you to start scratching, making your skin more inflamed, making your skin itch even more, making you scratch some more. Stop this vicious cycle with the Teenage and Adult Rash Relief. You have essential oils that stop the itch, clean and disinfect the area, and soothe the skin.

Teenage and Adult Rash Relief

12 drops Chamomile

15 drops Lavender

4 drops Peppermint

12 drops Tea Tree

> Mix all the oils together in a dark glass container.
>
> Put 22 drops of the blended oils in 8 ounces of water in a spray bottle. When you get a rash, spray the area with this blend, then let air dry.
>
> Add 30 drops of the essential oils to 4 ounces of base lotion or 4 tablespoons of carrier oil (any oil listed in the "Carrier Oils" chapter). Apply a small amount of the blend to the affected area 4 to 6 times a day until the rash heals. You can expect relief within 1 - 3 days.

Sometimes a rash causes the skin to become inflamed. The anti-inflammatory properties of Yarrow and Chamomile will help reduce the swelling, soothe the skin, and reduce your desire to scratch.

Rash Inflammation Treatment

20 drops Chamomile

16 drops Lavender

10 drops Yarrow

Mix all the oils together in a dark glass container.

Put 22 drops of the blended oils in 8 ounces of water in a spray bottle. When you get a rash, spray the area with this blend, then let air dry.

Add 30 drops of the essential oils to 4 ounces of base lotion or 4 tablespoons of carrier oil (any oil listed in the "Carrier Oils" chapter). Apply a small amount of the blend to the affected area 4 to 6 times a day until the rash heals. You can expect relief within 1 - 3 days.

Scar Tissue and Stretch Marks

"And not till the wound heals and the scar disappears, do we begin to discover where we are."

Thoreau

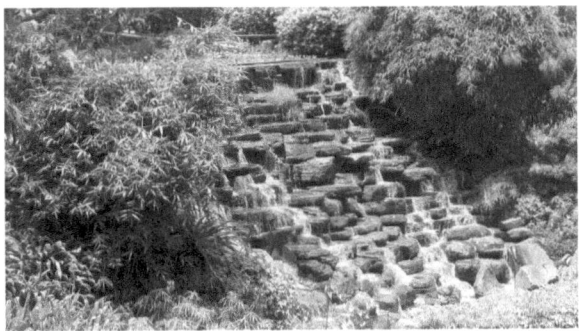

Finding who we really are, as Thoreau suggests, seems like a lifelong journey for many of us. Along the way we might get a scar here or a stretch mark there. If we are really lucky in life, these are only surface injuries. When they appear you can use essential oils to help heal them.

Scars result when the skin repairs wounds caused by accident, disease, or surgery. They are a natural part of the healing process. The more the skin is damaged and the longer it takes to heal, the greater the chance of a noticeable scar. Typically, a scar may appear redder and thicker at first, and then gradually fade. Many actively healing scars that seem unsightly at three months may heal nicely if given more time.

Stretch marks occur in the middle layer of skin known as the dermis. This layer is elastic and allows skin to retain its shape. When the dermis is constantly stretched over time, the skin becomes less elastic and the connective fibers break. The result is the markings we know as stretch marks which reveal colored skin marks on your body that seem to get brighter and then, over time, become less noticeable. Stretch marks can appear anywhere on the body where the skin has been stretched (often as a result of weight gain), such as abdomen, breasts, upper arms, thighs, and buttocks. They have no negative impact on your health; they are just unsightly.

In just about every section in this book, I have told you what you can do to prevent a certain ailment. There isn't much you can do to prevent scars and stretch marks, unless you want to live in a bubble, so take your licks and let aromatherapy help you fight back.

Essential Oil Blends

The best essential oils for healing your skin are: Carrot, Chamomile, Lavender, Patchouli, and Tea Tree. Refer to the "Essential Oil Chart" to learn about any contraindications, warnings, or cautions about using essential oils.

Scars and stretch marks don't appear overnight; therefore, they are not going to disappear overnight. I have successfully treated people who have had stretch marks for as many as seventeen years, but it took a commitment of 8 months to repair the skin to the point where the appearance of the stretch mark was gone. I know that you have surgical solutions that may give you quicker results, but I want you to have the choice of resolving the issue non-invasively and naturally.

Massage any of the following blends into the scarred area or the stretch marks. Apply the selected blend a minimum of twice daily for at least 3 months. By then you should see the scar tissue or stretch marks diminishing. Continue to use the blend at least twice a day to achieve your desired results. You can use the blend from 4 to 6 times a day until the visual appearance of scars or stretch marks diminish.

Scar Tissue Tightener

5 drops Carrot

10 drops Geranium

10 drops Lavender

5 drops Tangerine

> Add all drops of the essential oils and 10 drops of Borage Seed oil to 4 ounces of base lotion or 4 tablespoons of carrier oil (any oil listed in the "Carrier Oils" chapter). Apply a small amount of the blend to the affected area.

You will see the most successful results when you switch between the Scar Tissue Tightener and the Scar Tissue Soother blends. Use the Tightener blend for a month, then switch to the Soother blend for a month. Repeat this cycle until the scars are gone. The Tangerine and Carrot essential oils in the Tightener blend reach deeply into the affected area and work with your body to increase the elasticity. The Sandalwood and Frankincense in the Soother blend offer skin rejuvenation.

Scar Tissue Soother

8 drops Cypress

10 drops Frankincense

10 drops Lavender

5 drops Sandalwood

> Add all drops of the essential oils to 4 ounces of base lotion or 4 tablespoons of carrier oil (any oil listed in the "Carrier Oils" chapter). Massage a small amount of the blend into the affected area.

Notice that the ingredients in the Stretch Mark Tightener and Scar Tissue Tightener are the same. If you think about it, you can see why you would use essential oils that penetrate deeply to improve elasticity and nourish the skin.

Note: All the essential oils used in the Stretch Mark blends are safe for pregnancy.

Stretch Marks Tightener

5 drops Carrot

10 drops Geranium

10 drops Lavender

5 drops Tangerine

> Add all drops of the essential oils and 10 drops of Borage Seed oil to 4 ounces of base lotion or 4 tablespoons of carrier oil (any oil listed in the "Carrier Oils" chapter). Apply a small amount of the blend to the affected area.

> This blend should be helpful in avoiding stretch marks if you begin using it during the first trimester of pregnancy and continue throughout your pregnancy.

I suggest to clients that they actually take pictures of the area before they start using the blend, after one month, two months, and so on. The picture gives you a clearer understanding of the progress you are making.

The Stretch Marks Soother blend contains essential oils designed to nurture the skin as it returns to a state of health. Switch between these two blends. Use the Tightener blend for a month, then switch to the Soother blend for a month. Then repeat the cycle until the stretch marks are gone.

Stretch Marks Soother

10 drops Frankincense

8 drops Geranium

10 drops Lavender

5 drops Myrrh

> Add all drops of the essential oils to 4 ounces of base lotion or 4 tablespoons of carrier oil (any oil listed in the "Carrier Oils" chapter). Apply a small amount of the blend to the affected area.

> This blend should be helpful in avoiding stretch marks if you begin using it during the first trimester of pregnancy and continue throughout your pregnancy.

Shaving and Razor Burn

"The pain passes, but the beauty remains."

Pierre Auguste Renoir

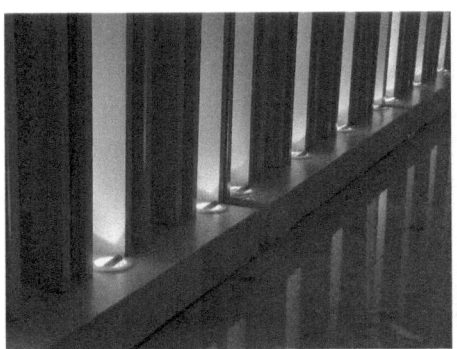

Face it; to feel well groomed, you have to spend some time shaving. It could be your underarms, your legs, or your face (if you are a man), but everywhere you shave you chance causing some sort of skin disturbance. Since I don't think the phrase, "No pain, no gain" refers to shaving, I have included several suggestions in this chapter to help the pain pass and allow the beauty to remain.

Shaving brings on many problems: dry and irritated skin, razor burn, shaving rash or itch, and razor bumps. Amazing that you would shave your skin on purpose when all that awaits you! But shave we do. We are in love with clean-shaven skin, whether it is on a man's face or on a woman's legs.

Applying too much pressure when you shave and using shaving products that contain synthetic fragrances, dyes, and alcohol can contribute to shaving problems.

When you shave, try to shave in the direction of the hair growth. While it may be tempting to shave against the grain, thinking you are getting a cleaner shave, you are actually cutting hair off just below the level of the skin. This causes the skin above to seal and then the hair causes bumps and redness in trying to break through the skin — razor bumps.

In his book, "The Wrinkle Cure," Dr. Nicholas Perricone suggests using alpha hydroxy acids to counteract razor bumps. Shaving experts also suggest that you use hot water while shaving to soften the hair and open the pores and to shave after a warm shower, not before.

Essential Oil Blends

The best essential oils for soothing and rejuvenating skin are Carrot, Chamomile, Geranium, Lavender, Lemon, Patchouli, Rosemary, and Thyme. Refer to the "Essential Oil Chart" for contraindications, warnings, or cautions about using essential oils.

If you are susceptible to shaving rash, shaving burn, or razor burn, it is a good idea to treat the skin immediately after shaving. Why wait for a rash to develop? *Ask any honest woman who has been shaving for more than ten years and she will admit that she has at one time wondered if she should just wear slacks.*

Shaving Treatment

5 drops Carrot

10 drops Lavender

8 drops Lemon

10 drops Rosemary

> As a daily shaving refresher, add all the essential oils and 2 teaspoons of either Witch Hazel or Apple Cider Vinegar to 8 ounces of water in a spray bottle. After shaving, spritz (3 – 5 squirts) the affected area, let air dry, then apply moisturizer. You can expect relief within 1 - 3 days.

Note: Avoid getting this into your eyes or other mucus membranes.

What you want after you shave is a toner (or after shave spritz) that will calm and deep clean your skin to avoid infections. Try this one.

Shaving Soother

10 drops Lavender

8 drops Lemon

10 drops Patchouli

5 drops Thyme

> As a daily shaving refresher, add all the essential oils and 2 teaspoons of either Witch Hazel or Apple Cider Vinegar to 8 ounces of water in a spray bottle. After shaving, spritz (3 – 5 squirts) the affected area, let air dry, then apply moisturizer. You can expect relief within 1 - 3 days.

Often times you will notice razor burn on skin that rubs against other skin such as your upper legs. Another key contributor to razor burn is sweating, such as under your arms. Make sure you keep this area as dry as possible. After using one of the razor burn blends, make sure you allow the area to dry completely.

My personal preference is to let the blend air-dry and then I apply a little bit of powder.

Razor Burn Relief

6 drops Chamomile

10 drops Geranium

10 drops Lavender

6 drops Lemon

> Mix all oils together. Add half this blend to a quart of water and use it to spritz the shaved area.
>
> For a more concentrated effect, add the other half of the blend to 2 tablespoons of lotion or carrier oil and massage the shaved area. Apply the blend 4 to 6 times a day until the burn subsides. You can expect relief within 1 - 3 days.

Note: Avoid getting this into your eyes or other mucus membranes.

If you have very sensitive skin, the Carrot essential oil in the Soothe the Burn blend is just what you need. *Here's the part about shaving that I don't understand. We shave our legs so that we give a good appearance. For me, the results are often legs covered with bandages – I don't find that very attractive, but I've never been the fashion guru anyway.*

Soothe the Burn

10 drops Carrot

15 drops Chamomile

10 drops Geranium

10 drops Lavender

Mix all the oils together in a dark glass container.

Add 20 drops of the blended oils to 8 ounces of water in a spray bottle. When you get razor burn, spray the area with this blend, then let air dry.

Note: Avoid getting this into your eyes or other mucus membranes.

Add 25 drops of the essential oils to 4 ounces of base lotion or 4 tablespoons of carrier oil (any oil listed in the "Carrier Oils" chapter). Apply a small amount of the blend to the affected area 4 to 6 times a day until the razor burn subsides. You can expect relief within 1 – 3 days.

Wrinkles

"Old age is no place for sissies."

Bette Davis

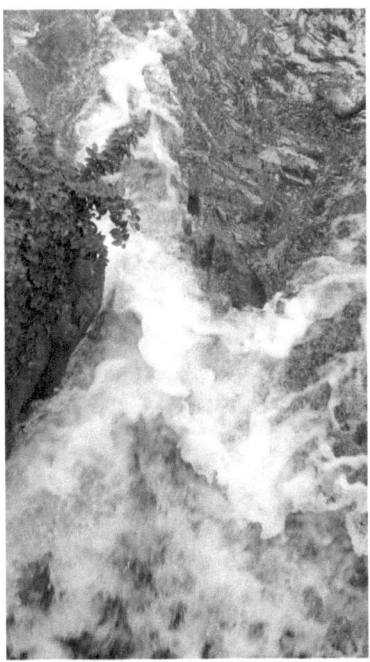

One morning you look into the mirror and you see a very (very) faint line. For a while, you may even tell yourself it's a smile line, an expression line. Finally, you will admit it – you have a wrinkle! Perhaps if you open your eyes wider, it will go away, perhaps if you don't smile or frown. Better to do something about it than to give up facial expressions.

Wrinkles are visible creases in the skin. Most wrinkles are associated with aging of the skin and skin structures, which is a natural process. While nothing can be done to decrease your skin's tendency to age — that is your genetic makeup — you can examine and deal with the many environmental factors that increase the rate at which skin ages. Environmental factors include poor nutrition, sun exposure, smoking, and drinking alcohol. *If you don't think the sun ages your skin, compare your face or hands with areas of your body that are protected from sunlight like your derriere.*

Because many skin changes are related to sun exposure, prevention is a lifelong process. Use a good quality sunscreen when outdoors, even in the winter. Wear protective clothing and hats as necessary. Good nutrition and adequate fluids are also helpful in keeping wrinkles at bay. Keep skin moist with lotions, and do not use soaps that are heavily perfumed. Moist skin is more comfortable and may heal better.

A good book on minimizing wrinkles is "The Wrinkle Cure" by Nicholas Perricone.

Essential Oil Blends

The best essential oils for battling wrinkles are Carrot, Clary Sage, Fennel, Frankincense, Geranium, Lavender, Myrrh, Patchouli, Rose, Rosemary, and Rosewood. *There are more expensive essential oils that you can use to improve your skin; however, I suggest you try these less expensive oils first and save the money to do something fun!* Refer to the "Essential Oil Chart" for contraindications, warnings, or cautions about using essential oils.

Use the following blends at least twice a day for 3 months. By that time you should see fewer wrinkles. Forever Young Skin was formulated for women in their mid-30s and above who have normal to dry skin.

Forever Young Skin

8 drops Cypress

10 drops Geranium

10 drops Lavender

5 drops Sandalwood

> Add all drops of the essential oils to 4 ounces of base lotion or 4 tablespoons of carrier oil (any oil listed in the "Carrier Oils" chapter). Cleanse your face. Using gentle upward strokes, apply a small amount of the blend to the face and neck area at least twice daily.

Smooth and Clear Skin was formulated for women in their mid-40s and above who have normal to oily skin.

I saw my daughter's kindergarten teacher after about five years. She asked in a whispered tone, "When did you get your face lift?" I held my head up high, put a large smile on my face, and clearly stated, "I didn't get a face lift. I've just been using essential oils." You know that she now uses this blend.

See the "Dry Skin" chapter to make moisturizers for dry facial skin.

Smooth and Clear Skin

5 drops Clary Sage

10 drops Frankincense

10 drops Lavender

8 drops Ylang Ylang

> Add all drops of the essential oils to 4 ounces of base lotion or 4 tablespoons of carrier oil (any oil listed in the "Carrier Oils" chapter). Cleanse your face. Using gentle upward strokes, apply a small amount of the blend to the face and neck area at least twice daily.

You can use the Day and Night Skin Care blend in a carrier oil for extra moisturizing at bedtime or mix it with water and witch hazel for a wonderful toner.

Day and Night Skin Care

8 drops Clary Sage

8 drops Fennel

6 drops Geranium

6 drops Lavender

> Mix the essential oils together. Use in one or both of the following ways:
>
> Add the blend to 2 tablespoons Sweet Almond Oil or Apricot Kernel oil. Massage this mixture on your clean face before bedtime.
>
> Add the blend to 4 ounces filtered water or spring water and 1 ounce witch hazel and use it as a toner, in the morning and at night.

For a quick treat for puffiness around the eyes, try the following blend.

Puffiness Reducer

2 drops Carrot

4 drops Lavender

2 drops Lemon

Dissolve the oils into 1 tablespoon of chilled witch hazel and 1 tablespoon cold water. Take a soft cotton towel and dip it into the blend. Gently apply a small amount of hazelnut oil to your closed eyes and then drape the towel over your closed eyes. Relax for a few minutes.

Emotional Support

What is scent therapy?

You would be amazed to learn how many colleges, universities, research facilities, and scientific resources are committed to the study of smell and taste. The research has provided some incredible insights. Of particular interest to us in the aromatherapy world, the research has shown that a particular fragrance or scent can elicit emotional reactions in humans.

There is a direct relationship between a smell and the experience associated with the smell. For example, you are on your honeymoon in Hawaii (any volunteers?). When you get off the plane, the temperature is in the mid 70's, the breeze is soft and balmy, there is a full moon, you can hear the ocean gently washing against the beach, and someone comes up to put a lei of plumeria flowers around your neck. Because of that one moment, in your mind the scent of plumeria will forever be associated with that totally awesome and romantic experience.

Whether it is 2 years later or 20 years later, all you have to do is smell plumeria to be immediately transported back to the wonderful emotional reactions you felt then. That, in a nutshell, is scent therapy.

Unfortunately, you may also have negative experiences associated with a fragrance. When you smell that scent again, you become emotional agitated, unhappy, frightened, or whatever negative emotion was originally associated with that experience.

The remainder of this section deals with:

- Anxiety, Fear, and Panic

- Concentration

- Depression

- Fatigue and Lethargy

- Grief

- Moodiness and Irritability

- Postpartum Depression

- Stress

Anxiety, Fear, and Panic

"Each problem that I solved became a rule which served afterwards to solve other problems."

Rene Descartes

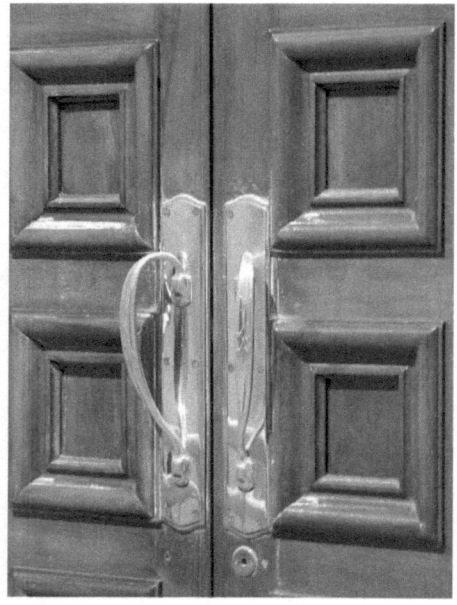

Learning from our mistakes without judging ourselves harshly is a wonderful idea. You can imagine that, even as a great philosopher and mathematician, Rene Descartes periodically suffered the angst of anxiety, fear, and panic. When these emotions attack, my gut feeling is to throw everything I can against them to offset them. Meditation, affirmations, brisk walks, essential oils, massage, and phone calls to a friend are part of my arsenal.

Anxiety is that tension that you might feel when you sense danger. Typically, the source of the danger is not known. Fear, on the other hand, is often associated with the same feeling of tension but you know the source of danger. Panic is sudden and exaggerated tension. It is normal to have some mild anxiety and fear present in our daily lives. Anxiety warns us and enables us to get ready for the 'fight or flight' response. However, heightened anxiety is emotionally painful. It disrupts a person's daily functioning.

In addition, you will experience physiological and biological changes; for example, your heart rate, blood pressure, hormonal levels, and adrenaline gland production go up. You may also experience twitching, trembling, muscle tension, headaches, irritability, sweating, hot flashes, lightheadedness, breathlessness, and nausea. You may have trouble falling asleep or staying asleep.

Anxiety and fear can become destructive and affect the quality of your life; making you feel out of control and possibly causing problems in your personal and professional relationships.

Both external and internal events can bring about these emotions. Both current events (such as an argument with your boss) and historical events (such as a childhood trauma) can trigger these emotions.

The healthiest way to deal with these emotions is to express them in a manner that helps resolve the underlying conflict. To do so, clear your mind, focus your thoughts, and create a viable plan. You may want to explore methods such as relaxation techniques, affirmations, reframing, humor, effective communication, and problem solving. You should also avoid caffeine — even one cup a day can bring on anxiety attacks. Try some caffeine-free peppermint tea instead. Cloves seem to have a calming action so try simmering some powdered clove in a pan of water on the stove to let the fragrance calm you. You can also bathe in clove tea to calm and sooth your body or, finally, drink a glass of warm milk to which you have added honey and ½ teaspoon powdered clove.

I recognize that each of these emotional conditions has distinct characteristics and associated physical symptoms; this chapter provides unique blends for each. My intent in combining these emotions in one category is for ease of reference for my readers.

Essential Oil Blends

The best essential oils for helping with emotions are:

- For Anxiety: Bergamot, Cedarwood, Chamomile, Clary Sage, Frankincense, Geranium, Juniper, Lavender, Mandarin, Neroli, Patchouli, Sandalwood, Vetiver, and Ylang Ylang.

- For Fear: Basil, Bergamot, Cedarwood, Chamomile, Clary Sage, Cypress, Frankincense, Lavender, Lemon, Neroli, Orange, Sandalwood, Vetiver, and Ylang Ylang.

- For Panic: Bergamot, Chamomile, Frankincense, Lavender, Marjoram, Rosemary, Spruce, and Ylang Ylang.

Refer to the "Essential Oil Chart" for contraindications, warnings, or cautions about using essential oils.

When treating anxiety, you want a blend that gives you a sense of peacefulness, comfort, and relaxation. Both of the following blends provide the chemical properties to meet those needs, so choose the one that resonates with you the most.

The night before my daughter was to give a speech to an auditorium of total strangers, I marveled at how soundly she could sleep while I was pacing the floor with anxiety. Thank goodness I used The Anxiety Relief – Option 2 and finally got a good night's sleep.

Refer to the "Emotional Support" section to learn more about scent therapy. Keeping scent therapy in mind, smell the individual essential oils in both the Option 1 and Option 2 blends. If a certain set of essential oils "resonates" with you, then these are the oils to use in treating your anxiety. Your body often wants to assist you in healing itself — listen closely and create the blend that most meets your needs.

For Anxiety

Anxiety Relief – Option 1

8 drops Bergamot

6 drops Cedarwood

4 drops Frankincense

8 drops Ylang Ylang

When you want to create a blend that you can smell and that absorbs into the skin, you can make a body oil or a body splash.

Add all of the essential oils to 2 tablespoons of carrier oil (any oil listed in the "Carrier Oils" chapter). Shake well and dab on your pulse points and at the base of your neck 4 to 6 times daily for the first week. Once you notice an improvement, you can reduce the applications to 2 to 3 times daily until your anxiety subsides.

To make a body splash, add all of the essential oils to 8 ounces of water in a spray bottle. Spritz (3 – 5 squirts) your upper body (upper chest and neck area) 4 to 6 times daily for the first week. Once you notice an improvement, you can reduce the applications to 2 to 3 times daily until your anxiety subsides.

Note: If you do not notice improvement at the end of the first week, continue to use the blend 4 to 6 times daily for up to 6 weeks. Progress with emotional concerns varies by individual.

You may want to continue to use the blend once daily simply to avoid the recurrence of anxiety.

Anxiety Relief – Option 2

6 drops Bergamot

6 drops Chamomile

6 drops Clary Sage

8 drops Ylang Ylang

When you want to create a blend that you can smell and that absorbs into the skin, you can make a body oil or a body splash.

Add all of the essential oils to 2 tablespoons of carrier oil (any oil listed in the "Carrier Oils" chapter). Shake well and dab on your pulse points and at the base of your neck 4 to 6 times daily for the first week. Once you notice an improvement, you can reduce the applications to 2 to 3 times daily until your anxiety subsides.

To make a body splash, add all of the essential oils to 8 ounces of water in a spray bottle. Spritz (3 – 5 squirts) your upper body (upper chest and neck area) 4 to 6 times daily for the first week. Once you notice an improvement, you can reduce the applications to 2 to 3 times daily until your anxiety subsides.

Note: If you do not notice improvement at the end of the first week, continue to use the blend 4 to 6 times daily for up to 6 weeks. Progress with emotional concerns varies by individual.

You may want to continue to use the blend once daily simply to avoid the recurrence of anxiety.

For Fear

When treating fear, you want a blend that provides a sense of safety, security, and protectiveness. All three of these blends provide the chemical properties to meet those needs, so choose the one that you like best.

Some research has shown that fear embeds itself into our bodies at the cellular level. Each year I can sense the anniversary of a traumatic event from my past because my body reacts with fear, increased heart rate, and a sense of gloom. Essential oils can really help.

Again, smell the essential oils individually and listen to your body's reaction to the oils. Then make a blend with the oils your body selected.

Fear Relief – Option 1

6 drops Chamomile

8 drops Lavender

6 drops Lemon

6 drops Orange

> When you want to create a blend that you can smell and that absorbs into the skin, you can make a body oil or a body splash.
>
> Add all of the essential oils to 2 tablespoons of carrier oil (any oil listed in the "Carrier Oils" chapter). Shake well and dab on your pulse points and at the base of your neck 4 to 6 times daily for the first week. Once you notice an improvement, you can reduce the applications to 2 to 3 times daily until your fear subsides.
>
> To make a body splash, add all of the essential oils to 8 ounces of water in a spray bottle. Spritz (3 – 5 squirts) your upper body (upper chest and neck area) 4 to 6 times daily for the first week. Once you notice an improvement, you can reduce the applications to 2 to 3 times daily until your fear subsides.

Note: If you do not notice improvement at the end of the first week, continue to use the blend 4 to 6 times daily for up to 6 weeks. Progress with emotional concerns varies by individual.

You may want to continue to use the blend once daily simply to avoid the recurrence of fear.

Fear Relief – Option 2

6 drops Bergamot

6 drops Chamomile

6 drops Clary Sage

8 drops Ylang Ylang

When you want to create a blend that you can smell and that absorbs into the skin, you can make a body oil or a body splash.

Add all of the essential oils to 2 tablespoons of carrier oil (any oil listed in the "Carrier Oils" chapter). Shake well and dab on your pulse points and at the base of your neck 4 to 6 times daily for the first week. Once you notice an improvement, you can reduce the applications to 2 to 3 times daily until your fear subsides.

To make a body splash, add all of the essential oils to 8 ounces of water in a spray bottle. Spritz (3 – 5 squirts) your upper body (upper chest and neck area) 4 to 6 times daily for the first week. Once you notice an improvement, you can reduce the applications to 2 to 3 times daily until your fear subsides.

Note: If you do not notice improvement at the end of the first week, continue to use the blend 4 to 6 times daily for up to 6 weeks. Progress with emotional concerns varies by individual.

You may want to continue to use the blend once daily simply to avoid the recurrence of fear.

Fear Relief – Option 3

6 drops Cypress

8 drops Juniper

6 drops Marjoram

6 drops Spruce

When you want to create a blend that you can smell and that absorbs into the skin, you can make a body oil or a body splash.

Add all of the essential oils to 2 tablespoons of carrier oil (any oil listed in the "Carrier Oils" chapter). Shake well and dab on your pulse points and at the base of your neck 4 to 6 times daily for the first week. Once you notice an improvement, you can reduce the applications to 2 to 3 times daily until your fear subsides.

To make a body splash, add all of the essential oils to 8 ounces of water in a spray bottle. Spritz (3 – 5 squirts) your upper body (upper chest and neck area) 4 to 6 times daily for the first week. Once you notice an improvement, you can reduce the applications to 2 to 3 times daily until your fear subsides.

Note: If you do not notice improvement at the end of the first week, continue to use the blend 4 to 6 times daily for up to 6 weeks. Progress with emotional concerns varies by individual.

You may want to continue to use the blend once daily simply to avoid the recurrence of fear.

For Panic

When treating panic, you want a blend that gives you a sense of self-control, calmness, and strength. Both of the following blends provide the chemical properties to meet those needs, so choose the one that you like best.

Panic Relief – Option 1

6 drops Bergamot

6 drops Chamomile

8 drops Lavender

6 drops Ylang Ylang

When you want to create a blend that you can smell and that absorbs into the skin, you can make a body oil or a body splash.

Add all of the essential oils to 2 tablespoons of carrier oil (any oil listed in the "Carrier Oils" chapter). Shake well and dab on your pulse points and at the base of your neck 4 to 6 times daily for the first week. Once you notice an improvement, you can reduce the applications to 2 to 3 times daily until your panic subsides.

To make a body splash, add all of the essential oils to 8 ounces of water in a spray bottle. Spritz (3 – 5 squirts) your upper body (upper chest and neck area) 4 to 6 times daily for the first week. Once you notice an improvement, you can reduce the applications to 2 to 3 times daily until your panic subsides.

Note: If you do not notice improvement at the end of the first week, continue to use the blend 4 to 6 times daily for up to 6 weeks. Progress with emotional concerns varies by individual.

You may want to continue to use the blend once daily simply to avoid the recurrence of panic.

Panic Relief – Option 2

8 drops Lavender

6 drops Marjoram

6 drops Rosemary

6 drops Spruce

> When you want to create a blend that you can smell and that absorbs into the skin, you can make a body oil or a body splash.
>
> Add all of the essential oils to 2 tablespoons of carrier oil (any oil listed in the "Carrier Oils" chapter). Shake well and dab on your pulse points and at the base of your neck 4 to 6 times daily for the first week. Once you notice an improvement, you can reduce the applications to 2 to 3 times daily until your panic subsides.
>
> To make a body splash, add all of the essential oils to 8 ounces of water in a spray bottle. Spritz (3 – 5 squirts) your upper body (upper chest and neck area) 4 to 6 times daily for the first week. Once you notice an improvement, you can reduce the applications to 2 to 3 times daily until your panic subsides.

Note: If you do not notice improvement at the end of the first week, continue to use the blend 4 to 6 times daily for up to 6 weeks. Progress with emotional concerns varies by individual.

You may want to continue to use the blend once daily simply to avoid the recurrence of panic.

Concentration

"The ability to concentrate and to use time well is everything."

Lee Iacocca

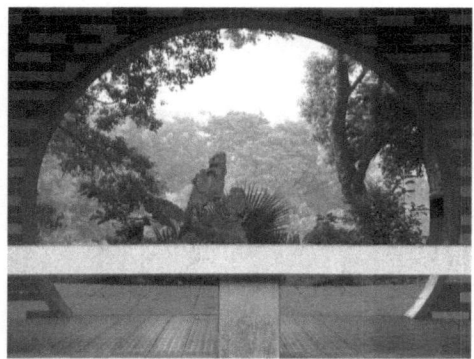

The ability to concentrate was only part of Lee's success, but I'm sure it was a large part. Concentration is something that impacts many parts of our lives, both personally and professionally. For those of us who require additional help with concentration, let me share a couple of my own personal suggestions. Write a plan with realistic reachable goals. Don't get involved with negative thoughts or feelings because you don't have a terrific concentration level. Work with what you've got and work around what you don't.

There is a lot written about the benefits of concentration. You receive great satisfaction when you are focused because typically you are more successful and able to work efficiently. You can see acts of concentration everywhere: from children working hard to write those first letters of their name to adults multi-tasking. Research has shown that people have varying degrees of concentration. Some people can focus with the music blaring. Others require absolute silence. Some people can talk on the phone, make dinner, and correct their child's spelling test all at the same time. Others can barely get through one task if they are interrupted. Finally, people feel differently about concentration. For those who can do it well, it doesn't seem like a big deal. For those who struggle with concentration, it can be a major stumbling block in their lives.

With all the research I did on concentration, I could not find one bit of information about what causes people to have varying abilities when it comes to concentration. Somewhat selfishly, since I am at the end of the spectrum that requires no interruptions, no music, and a single-minded attack on any project I am given, I was hoping to find a cause like genetics. Fortunately, research has suggested that essential oils can enhance your powers of concentration.

Essential Oil Blends

The citrus oils help you focus and are uplifting. This includes Bergamot, Lemon, Lemongrass, and Orange. Other oils that help your concentration are Basil, Cardamom, Cedarwood, Eucalyptus, Peppermint, and Rosemary. Refer to the "Essential Oil Chart" for contraindications, warnings, or cautions about using essential oils.

Refer to the "Emotional Support" section to learn more about scent therapy. Diffusing essential oils in your office, study room, or den is a great way to aid your concentration. Use either of these first two blends:

Aromatic Concentration Potpourri

5 drops Rosemary

> Mix lemon rinds, apple peels, and Rosemary in 16 ounces of water. Pour into either a potpourri pot or saucepan and apply low heat. You'll love how you are able to remain calm and focused.

Perhaps you prefer the convenience of a room spray. It's quick and you can take it with you. This is perfect for the students in your family.

Concentration Room Spray

4 drops Basil

2 drop Eucalyptus

8 drops Lavender

4 drops Orange

4 drops Rosemary

> Mix all the oils together. Add the essential oils to 16 ounces of water and use as a room spray before you sit down to study. Refresh the room from time to time as you study.

If you would rather apply the essential oil blend to your body so as not to disturb others that might be sharing a study area with you, try the Personal Concentration Blend.

I use this blend when I work in my daughter's school because, in addition to helping me with my concentration, it also contains essential oils that help keep germs away.

Personal Concentration Blend

6 drops Cedarwood

6 drops Eucalyptus

8 drops Lavender

6 drops Lemon

When you want to create a blend that you can smell and that absorbs into the skin, you can make a body oil or a body splash.

Add all of the essential oils to 2 tablespoons of carrier oil (any oil listed in the "Carrier Oils" chapter). Shake well and dab on your pulse points and at the base of your neck 4 to 6 times daily for the first week. If you notice an improvement, you can reduce the applications to 2 to 3 times daily until you feel your brain sharpen.

To make a body splash, add all of the essential oils to 8 ounces of water in a spray bottle. Spritz (3 – 5 squirts) your upper body (upper chest and neck area) 4 to 6 times daily for the first week. If you notice an improvement, you can reduce the applications to 2 to 3 times daily until you feel your brain sharpen.

Note: If you do not notice improvement at the end of the first week, continue to use the blend 4 to 6 times daily for up to 6 weeks. Progress with concentration varies by individual.

You may want to continue to use the blend once daily simply to feel sharper.

Another effective way to improve your concentration for studying or memorization is to inhale the essential oils directly.

If you feel anxious or tense when you try to concentrate, like before giving a speech or while studying for an important exam, try the Focus and Concentration blend.

I worked with a high school debate team, and this blend helped them focus and concentrate, and it also gave them a sense of confidence and purpose.

Focus and Concentration

6 drops Juniper

8 drops Lavender

6 drops Lemon

6 drops Peppermint

When you want to create a blend that you can smell and that absorbs into the skin, you can make a body oil or a body splash.

Add all of the essential oils to 2 tablespoons of carrier oil (any oil listed in the "Carrier Oils" chapter). Shake well and dab on your pulse points and at the base of your neck 4 to 6 times daily for the first week. If you notice an improvement, you can reduce the applications to 2 to 3 times daily until you feel sharper.

To make a body splash, add all of the essential oils to 8 ounces of water in a spray bottle. Spritz (3 – 5 squirts) your upper body (upper chest and neck area) 4 to 6 times daily for the first week. If you notice an improvement, you can reduce the applications to 2 to 3 times daily until you feel sharper.

Note: If you do not notice improvement at the end of the first week, continue to use the blend 4 to 6 times daily for up to 6 weeks. Progress with concentration varies by individual.

You may want to continue to use the blend once daily simply to feel sharper.

Another effective way to improve your concentration for studying or memorization is to inhale the essential oils directly.

Sometimes (perhaps often with our hectic schedules) you need extra help to concentrate in your car. I have found just a drop of Rosemary on a tissue when I'm driving helps me stay alert and focused.

Depression

"The best cure for worry, depression, melancholy, brooding, is to go deliberately forth and try to lift with one's sympathy the gloom of somebody else."

Arnold Bennett

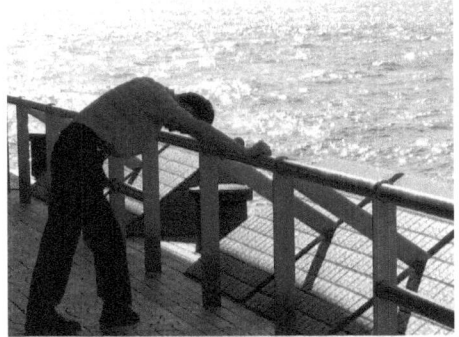

Who knows if the English novelist Arnold Bennett ever experienced depression, but his suggestion to move forward with a positive outlook makes great sense.

There is a significant amount of research done on depression. Feelings of sadness, helplessness, guilt, worthlessness, and pessimism are the primary symptoms. In addition, sufferers may experience lack of interest in life's pleasures, loss of concentration, indecision, guilt, slower physical and mental responses, and thoughts of suicide. Such negative thoughts and feelings make some people feel like giving up. It is important to realize that these negative views are part of the depression and, typically, do not accurately reflect the actual circumstances. Negative thinking fades as treatment begins to take effect.

Physical symptoms, such as weight loss or weight gain, headaches, digestive disorders, and chronic pain, may also indicate depression. Women experience depression about twice as often as men. For short-term depressive states, it might be helpful to:

- Break large tasks into small ones, set some priorities, and do *what* you can *as* you can.

- Try to be with other people and to confide in someone.

- Participate in activities that may make you feel better, including mild exercise.

- Expect your mood to improve gradually, not immediately. Feeling better takes time. If you are not sensing improvement after two weeks, consult your doctor to explore options.

- Don't make important decisions until the depression has lifted.

You can also treat yourself to natural healing support by using blends made of essential oils. Not only will the natural chemicals found in the plants help equalize your hormonal levels, but also the soothing scents can help lift your spirits. If your depression lasts for more than a couple of weeks or if you are experiencing suicidal thoughts, immediately consult your physician.

Essential Oil Blends

Essential oils that are helpful with depression are: Chamomile, Geranium, Patchouli, and Ylang Ylang for weepiness; Clary Sage,

Cypress, Grapefruit, and Rosemary for lethargy; Cedar, Sandalwood, and Vetiver for emotional release; and Bergamot, Chamomile, Cypress, Marjoram, and Rosemary for emotional exhaustion. Refer to the "Essential Oil Chart" for contraindications, warnings, or cautions about using essential oils.

When treating depression, you want a blend that gives you a sense of contentment, joy, and satisfaction. Refer to the "Emotional Support" section to learn more about scent therapy.

While a famous song laments that "I can't get noooo satisfaction," you can with one of these blends.

Depression Relief

6 drops Frankincense

6 drops Geranium

8 drops Lavender

6 drops Lemon

When you want to create a blend that you can smell and that absorbs into the skin, you can make a body oil or a body splash.

Add all of the essential oils to 2 tablespoons of carrier oil (any oil listed in the "Carrier Oils" chapter). Shake well and dab on your pulse points and at the base of your neck 4 to 6 times daily for the first week. If you notice an improvement, you can reduce the applications to 2 to 3 times daily until your depression subsides.

To make a body splash, add all of the essential oils to 8 ounces of water in a spray bottle. Spritz (3 – 5 squirts) your upper body (upper chest and neck area) 4 to 6 times daily for the first week. If you notice an improvement, you can reduce the applications to 2 to 3 times daily until your depression subsides.

Note: If you do not notice improvement at the end of the first week, continue to use the blend 4 to 6 times daily for up to 6 weeks. Progress with emotional concerns varies by individual.

You may want to continue to use the blend once daily simply to avoid the recurrence of depression.

Depression Support

8 drops Grapefruit

6 drops Lemon

6 drops Orange

6 drops Sandalwood

When you want to create a blend that you can smell and that absorbs into the skin, you can make a body oil or a body splash.

Add all of the essential oils to 2 tablespoons of carrier oil (any oil listed in the "Carrier Oils" chapter). Shake well and dab on your pulse points and at the base of your neck 4 to 6 times daily for the first week. If you notice an improvement, you can reduce the applications to 2 to 3 times daily until your depression subsides.

To make a body splash, add all of the essential oils to 8 ounces of water in a spray bottle. Spritz (3 – 5 squirts) your upper body (upper chest and neck area) 4 to 6 times daily for the first week. If you notice an improvement, you can reduce the applications to 2 to 3 times daily until your depression subsides.

Note: If you do not notice improvement at the end of the first week, continue to use the blend 4 to 6 times daily for up to 6 weeks. Progress with emotional concerns varies by individual.

You may want to continue to use the blend once daily simply to avoid the recurrence of depression.

Fatigue and Lethargy

"The significant problems we face cannot be solved at the same level of thinking we were at when we created them."

Albert Einstein

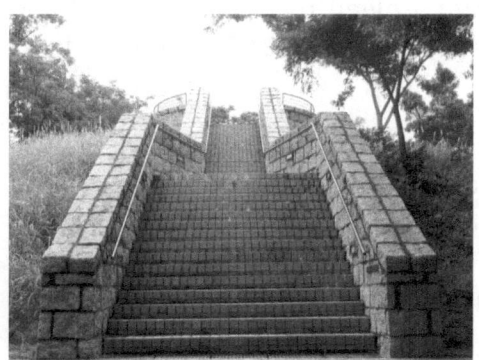

Einstein always had a way of saying something that makes you have to read it several times to get the point. Here he suggests that we cannot solve a problem while we are still experiencing the emotions that existed when the problem occurred. Take a deep breath, count to ten, find a new emotional state — one that is more objective — to focus on a solution to your problem. Great advice, once you get the message, but not always easy to do when you are tired or lethargic.

Occasional fatigue because you are not sleeping well or are under stress is not uncommon. Making sure you are eating well, exercising, and getting sufficient sleep is probably the best way to deal with occasional fatigue.

While fatigue may have a direct correlation to lack of sleep or a specific stressor, lethargy does not have that same one-to-one relationship with outside influences. Many people who feel lethargic can't pinpoint the cause of their emotional state, and thus frequently struggle with additional stress. They believe if they can't figure out what caused them to feel lethargic, then they can't figure out how to fix it. Lethargy can impact your energy levels throughout the day. You wake up feeling lethargic, never get your usual feeling of "get up and go," and by the end of the day you just feel drained.

If you experience fatigue or lethargy for any period of time you should consult your doctor. You may feel hesitant to seek a doctor's opinion because you want to avoid medication you believe the doctor will prescribe. Don't let that bias stand in your way. Your doctor can run simple tests to rule out physical or chemical causes of your current mental state. Get as much information as you can from your doctor and let her/him know that you want to resolve this issue with more natural solutions. If you get a clean "bill of health" from your doctor, you are still in control of the course of action to take. Your doctor can, however, make you aware of some of your options, including prescribed medication, over-the-counter medication, and other more natural solutions that previous patients have had success with.

Essential Oil Blends

The best essential oils for your emotional needs are grouped accordingly to symptom. For fatigue, try Clary Sage, Grapefruit, Lavender, Lemon, Marjoram, Orange, Peppermint, and Rosemary. For lethargy, try Bergamot, Chamomile, Cypress, Fennel, Geranium, Ginger, Lemon, Orange, Sandalwood, and Ylang Ylang. Refer to the "Essential Oil Chart" for contraindications, warnings, or cautions about using essential oils.

I recognize that fatigue and lethargy have distinct characteristics and associated physical symptoms, so I offer unique blends for each. I have combined them in the same chapter for ease of reference for my readers.

Refer to the "Emotional Support" section to learn more about scent therapy. *I love the smell of freshly cut grass. It reminds me of long summer days of my childhood. Just driving by someone else's freshly cut grass can make me remember summer vacations spent reading under our big maple tree or swinging as high as I could on a dare. For someone else the smell of freshly cut grass might be a negative – too many days taken up with chores of mowing the lawn or allergies!*

For Fatigue

In treating fatigue, you want a blend that provides an uplifting sense of focus, purpose, and direction without making you feel buzzed or over stimulated. Both of the following blends provide aromatherapeutic properties than can help you meet those goals, so choose the one that resonates for you the most.

Relief from Fatigue

5 drops Clary Sage

15 drops Lavender

10 drops Lemon

> Combine the essential oils with 1 cup of water in a spray bottle. Spray your upper body or into the air for a sweet, slightly energizing boost.

Fatigue Treatment

8 drops Lavender

2 drop Lemon

6 drops Orange

4 drops Rosemary

> Mix the oils together and use them in one of the following ways:
>
> Mix oils in 1 cup water and spray your work environment.
>
> Mix the above oils in 2 tablespoons carrier oil for an after-bath or after-shower oil to use in the morning. Rub the oil onto still-moist skin to seal in moisture and energize your day.

For Lethargy

To treat lethargy, you want a blend that gives you a sense of hopefulness, resolution, and persistence. The following blends provide the aromatherapeutic properties that can help you meet those goals. Remember what we know about scent therapy and let your nose and experiences guide you to the blend that makes most sense for you.

Lethargy Treatment

8 drops Bergamot

6 drops Geranium

6 drops Orange

6 drops Ylang Ylang

> When you want to create a blend that you can smell and that absorbs into the skin, you can make a body oil or a body splash.
>
> Add all of the essential oils to 2 tablespoons of carrier oil (any oil listed in the "Carrier Oils" chapter). Shake well and dab on your pulse points and at the base of your neck 4 to 6 times daily for the first week. Once you notice an improvement, you can reduce the applications to 2 to 3 times daily until your anxiety subsides.
>
> To make a body splash, add all of the essential oils to 8 ounces of water in a spray bottle. Spritz (3 – 5 squirts) your upper body (upper chest and neck area) 4 to 6 times daily for the first week. Once you notice an improvement, you can reduce the applications to 2 to 3 times daily until your anxiety subsides.

Note: If you do not notice improvement at the end of the first week, continue to use the blend 4 to 6 times daily for up to 6 weeks. Progress with emotional concerns varies by individual.

You may want to continue to use the blend once daily simply to avoid the recurrence of lethargy.

Relief from Lethargy

6 drops Cypress

6 drops Ginger

8 drops Orange

6 drops Sandalwood

> When you want to create a blend that you can smell and that absorbs into the skin, you can make a body oil or a body splash.
>
> Add all of the essential oils to 2 tablespoons of carrier oil (any oil listed in the "Carrier Oils" chapter). Shake well and dab on your pulse points and at the base of your neck 4 to 6 times daily for the first week. Once you notice an improvement, you can reduce the applications to 2 to 3 times daily until your anxiety subsides.
>
> To make a body splash, add all of the essential oils to 8 ounces of water in a spray bottle. Spritz (3 – 5 squirts) your upper body (upper chest and neck area) 4 to 6 times daily for the first week. Once you notice an improvement, you can reduce the applications to 2 to 3 times daily until your anxiety subsides.

Note: If you do not notice improvement at the end of the first week, continue to use the blend 4 to 6 times daily for up to 6 weeks. Progress with emotional concerns varies by individual.

You may want to continue to use the blend once daily simply to avoid the recurrence of lethargy.

The Emotional Energy Booster blend is wonderful because it contains hormone regulators, natural anti-depressants, and other soothing ingredients.

Emotional Energy Booster

8 drops Chamomile

7 drops Clary Sage

7 drops Fennel

8 drops Geranium

> When you want to create a blend that you can smell and that absorbs into the skin, you can make a body oil or a body splash.
>
> Add all of the essential oils to 2 tablespoons of carrier oil (any oil listed in the "Carrier Oils" chapter). Shake well and dab on your pulse points and at the base of your neck 4 to 6 times daily for the first week. Once you notice an improvement, you can reduce the applications to 2 to 3 times daily until your anxiety subsides.
>
> To make a body splash, add all of the essential oils to 8 ounces of water in a spray bottle. Spritz (3 – 5 squirts) your upper body (upper chest and neck area) 4 to 6 times daily for the first week. Once you notice an improvement, you can reduce the applications to 2 to 3 times daily until your anxiety subsides.

Note: If you do not notice improvement at the end of the first week, continue to use the blend 4 to 6 times daily for up to 6 weeks. Progress with emotional concerns varies by individual.

> You may want to continue to use the blend once daily simply to avoid the recurrence of lethargy.

Grief

"If you can't get rid of the skeleton in your closet, you'd best teach it to dance."

George Bernard Shaw

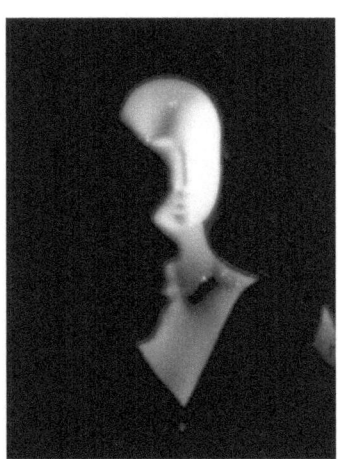

Susan's mother passed away; Eric was in the middle of a divorce; Hank's hunting dog died; Janet's home caught fire and several irreplaceable photographs and items were destroyed. All of these individuals have experienced grief, although it was brought about by very different events. Grief is a sense of intense sorrow. It goes beyond sadness. You feel it in the pit of your stomach and in the core of your soul. The impact of grief can influence every aspect of your physical, mental, and emotional well-being.

Many psychologists believe that grief is a normal, healthy response to loss. As you face a loss, you may have different feelings at different times. These feelings may include shock, denial, anger, guilt, sadness and acceptance. Healing from a loss involves coming to terms with the loss and the meaning of the loss in your life. People travel through this process at their own pace. Don't expect that within a certain period of time you will have worked completely through these feelings. If you're having trouble getting through the process, ask for help. People who can help include friends, family, clergy, a counselor or therapist, support groups, and your family doctor.

Try to maintain your daily routine, get enough sleep, eat a well-balanced diet, exercise, avoid alcohol, and do not put additional pressure on yourself.

If you are experiencing symptoms such as dizziness, disorientation, hyperventilating, shortness of breath, and other life-disrupting feelings, you should contact your doctor to get assistance right away.

Essential oil therapy can be very effective in helping you work through your grief. This additional natural support will not interfere with other healing strategies and can offer you safe and effective benefits.

Essential Oil Blends

Essential oils such as Bergamot, Chamomile, Cypress, Frankincense, and Nutmeg help ease feelings of grief. Clary Sage and Lavender offer a calming environment. Eucalyptus, Juniper, and Lemon offer a supportive and encouraging environment. Vetiver helps you express grief. Refer to the "Essential Oil Chart" for contraindications, warnings, or cautions about using essential oils.

You can use multiple essential oil blends to treat the same ailment. You might want to use the Grief Relief blend in the evening to provide a calming respite from grief. Refer to the "Emotional Support" section to learn more about scent therapy.

When my mother passed away in 2000, I knew that I would forever miss our daily phone calls, her practical words of encouragement, and her arms that were always open to me. I personally used these blends to support my journey through grief.

Grief Relief

8 drops Bergamot

6 drops Chamomile

6 drops Clary Sage

6 drops Lavender

When you want to create a blend that you can smell and that absorbs into the skin, you can make a body oil or a body splash.

Add all of the essential oils to 2 tablespoons of carrier oil (any oil listed in the "Carrier Oils" chapter). Shake well and dab on your pulse points and at the base of your neck 4 to 6 times daily for the first week. Once you notice an improvement, you can reduce the applications to 2 to 3 times daily until your anxiety subsides.

To make a body splash, add all of the essential oils to 8 ounces of water in a spray bottle. Spritz (3 – 5 squirts) your upper body (upper chest and neck area) 4 to 6 times daily for the first week. Once you notice an improvement, you can reduce the applications to 2 to 3 times daily until your anxiety subsides.

Note: If you do not notice improvement at the end of the first week, continue to use the blend 4 to 6 times daily for up to 6 weeks. Progress with emotional concerns varies by individual.

When you are feeling better, you may discontinue using the blend. However, start using the blend again whenever those feelings of grief recur.

The Grief Support blend is wonderful to use during the day because in addition to providing assistance for grief, it also has essential oils that help invigorate you and keep your physical body healthy while you heal emotionally.

Grief Support

6 drops Eucalyptus

6 drops Juniper

8 drops Lavender

6 drops Lemon

When you want to create a blend that you can smell and that absorbs into the skin, you can make a body oil or a body splash.

Add all of the essential oils to 2 tablespoons of carrier oil (any oil listed in the "Carrier Oils" chapter). Shake well and dab on your pulse points and at the base of your neck 4 to 6 times daily for the first week. Once you notice an improvement, you can reduce the applications to 2 to 3 times daily until your anxiety subsides.

To make a body splash, add all of the essential oils to 8 ounces of water in a spray bottle. Spritz (3 – 5 squirts) your upper body (upper chest and neck area) 4 to 6 times daily for the first week. Once you notice an improvement, you can reduce the applications to 2 to 3 times daily until your anxiety subsides.

Note: If you do not notice improvement at the end of the first week, continue to use the blend 4 to 6 times daily for up to 6 weeks. Progress with emotional concerns varies by individual.

When you are feeling better, you may discontinue using the blend. However, start using the blend again whenever those feelings of grief recur.

Moodiness and Irritability

"Whether you think that you can, or that you can't, you are usually right."

Henry Ford

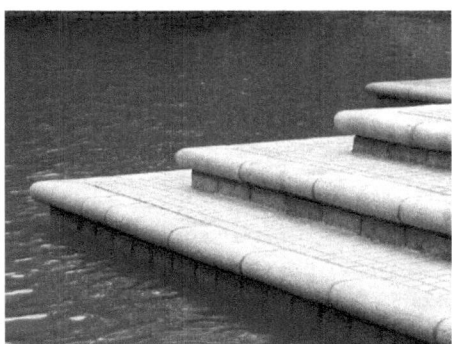

"I feel like I'm the ball in a brutal tennis match," said Patrick, a 15-year old high school student who demonstrated an unusual amount of awareness of his moodiness. Feeling that he was trapped and not in control of these emotions only made the problem worse. When you think that you are irritable, you are usually right, so let essential oils help.

Moods span the full spectrum of emotions, and we all experience moods throughout the day. General moodiness moves into irritability when you are being overly sensitive to stimulation. The primary goal of someone who wants to deal with moodiness is actually to find a balance among her or his many moods. Take a moment, clear your head, and gently focus on what is at the core of the particular mood. Once you identify the mood, you can often develop a balancing strategy, such as visualization, affirmations, or deep breathing. In many cases, simple identification of the source of a mood helps you feel more even keeled. You can also help yourself by avoiding stimulants such as nicotine, alcohol, and caffeine; and finding the time to rest and regroup.

Research shows that rapid fluctuations in hormones are accompanied by moodiness, irritability, impulsivity, aggression, and depression. Beyond the influence of hormones upon mood, there are other causes or imbalances that need to be addressed. If you or someone you know is in a depressed mood that lasts for two weeks or more, speak with your doctor or get outside help.

When dealing with moodiness and irritability in our children, many child psychologists and other professionals who deal with adolescents suggest that we parents provide consistent parameters in which a child can feel safe. Try to avoid getting in arguments when your child is acting particularly moody. Be patient, walk away, or ignore it. It is very difficult for someone to fight with you if you won't fight back.

In addition to these strategies, essential oil therapy can help equalize hormonal fluctuations and offer relaxing and calming properties, safely and effectively.

And remember, happiness is a mood too!

Essential Oil Blends

Essential oils that are effective in aiding emotional balancing are: Lemon, Peppermint, Pine, and Tea Tree to release negative feelings; Black Pepper, Cedarwood, Nutmeg, and Rosewood to expel negativity; Frankincense, Grapefruit, Lavender, and Rosemary for a feeling of acceptance; and Bergamot, Geranium, Marjoram, and Patchouli for a sense of assurance.

For Irritability: Chamomile (both German and Roman), Clary Sage, Cypress, Lavender, Neroli, Orange, Patchouli, Tangerine, Vetiver, and Ylang Ylang can all be helpful. Refer to the "Essential Oil Chart" for contraindications, warnings, or cautions about using essential oils.

The All Purpose Spray is great for a couple of reasons. The healthy antiseptic and antibacterial properties of this blend give you a jump on keeping your physical health strong while your emotional health is improving. The uplifting fragrance and chemical properties of these oils provide overall encouragement and confidence to help achieve good mental health.

All Purpose Spray

4 drops Lavender

2 drops Peppermint

2 drops Tea Tree

Mix oils in 2 cups of water. Spray throughout the house.

If you are the spouse or parent of a "grouch" you may want to diffuse the Grouch Prevention blend by putting 9 drops of the blend in a cup of water in a potpourri pot or by putting the entire blend in a cool mist vaporizer to carry the effective oils throughout the room. *One client said to me, "It's incredible what this stuff does, not only for my cranky teenager, but for his cranky parents as well."*

Grouch Prevention

2 drops Lavender

2 drops Lemon

2 drops Peppermint

6 drops Rosemary

6 drops Tea Tree

> Mix all oils together. Use the blend in one of these ways:
>
> Add all oils to 8 ounces of water and spray the air around the potential grouch as soon as he or she (or you) get up.
>
> Mix the essential oils in 2 tablespoons of any vegetable oil to use as a body oil after showering.

Whether it is the hormonal balancing effect of these oils or the more feminine fragrance of the blend, women prefer the For Her blend.

Feeling Good Body Splash – For Her

2 drops Bergamot

2 drops Lavender

2 drops Lemon

> Mix all oils in 8 ounces of water and use as a body splash to enhance your mood.

In addition to the following blend being great for treating moodiness, several of my clients use it as a refreshing and healthy aftershave. If you want additional antiseptic assistance for your face after shaving, add 2 ounces of witch hazel to the For Him blend.

Feeling Good Body Splash – For Him

10 drops Bergamot

11 drops Black Pepper

4 drops Cedarwood

3 drops Nutmeg

4 drops Rosewood

> Add all the essential oils to 2 cups water for an air spray or a body splash.

For Irritability

Refer to the "Emotional Support" section to learn more about scent therapy. When treating irritability, you want a blend that provides relaxation, serenity, and tranquility. Both of these blends have the chemical properties to meet those goals, so choose the one that resonates with you the most. *Being irritable, especially when you can't figure out what is causing it, is draining. When a nice warm bath or a long walk doesn't work, I get out my essential oils.*

Irritability Relief – Option 1

8 drops Lavender

6 drops Orange

6 drops Patchouli

6 drops Tangerine

When you want to create a blend that you can smell and that absorbs into the skin, you can make a body oil or a body splash.

Add all of the essential oils to 2 tablespoons of carrier oil (any oil listed in the "Carrier Oils" chapter). Shake well and dab on your pulse points and at the base of your neck 4 to 6 times daily for the first week. Once you notice an improvement, you can reduce the applications to 2 to 3 times daily until your anxiety subsides.

To make a body splash, add all of the essential oils to 8 ounces of water in a spray bottle. Spritz (3 – 5 squirts) your upper body (upper chest and neck area) 4 to 6 times daily for the first week. Once you notice an improvement, you can reduce the applications to 2 to 3 times daily until your anxiety subsides.

Note: If you do not notice improvement at the end of the first week, continue to use the blend 4 to 6 times daily for up to 6 weeks. Progress with emotional concerns varies by individual.

You may want to continue to use the blend once daily simply to avoid the recurrence of irritability.

Irritability Relief – Option 2

6 drops Chamomile

6 drops Clary Sage

8 drops Lavender

6 drops Vetiver

> When you want to create a blend that you can smell and that absorbs into the skin, you can make a body oil or a body splash.
>
> Add all of the essential oils to 2 tablespoons of carrier oil (any oil listed in the "Carrier Oils" chapter). Shake well and dab on your pulse points and at the base of your neck 4 to 6 times daily for the first week. Once you notice an improvement, you can reduce the applications to 2 to 3 times daily until your anxiety subsides.
>
> To make a body splash, add all of the essential oils to 8 ounces of water in a spray bottle. Spritz (3 – 5 squirts) your upper body (upper chest and neck area) 4 to 6 times daily for the first week. Once you notice an improvement, you can reduce the applications to 2 to 3 times daily until your anxiety subsides.

Note: If you do not notice improvement at the end of the first week, continue to use the blend 4 to 6 times daily for up to 6 weeks. Progress with emotional concerns varies by individual.

> You may want to continue to use the blend once daily simply to avoid the recurrence of irritability.

Postpartum Depression

"If you are going through hell, keep going."

Sir Winston Churchill

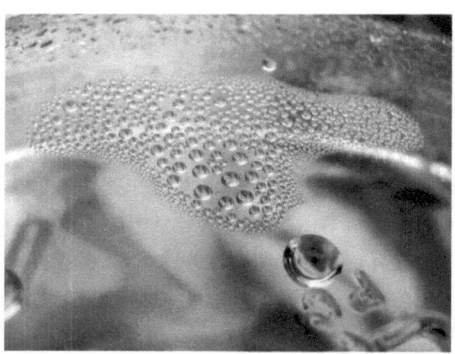

Sir Winston Churchill could never fully understand postpartum depression, but this emotional ailment has been around since way before his time. To follow his suggestion, this does feel like hell, and you need to keep going.

While it is common for women to have mood swings for up to 10 days after delivering a baby, if symptoms of sadness, irritability, and loss of appetite persist, you may have postpartum depression. Must every new mother experience a loss of interest or pleasure in life, less motivation, feelings of worthlessness or worry? No, but if you have had postpartum depression with previous births, general non-pregnancy related depression, severe PMS, difficult personal relationships, or too much stress, then you are a likely candidate for the "baby blues." The exact cause isn't known but hormone levels that change during pregnancy and right after childbirth may produce chemical changes in the brain that play a part in causing depression.

Other symptoms to keep an eye on are sleeping more than usual, or feeling worthless, hopeless, or overly guilty. Don't let these feelings continue, hoping that they will just pass. You can help yourself during this time by finding someone to talk to, getting help with chores and errands, taking time for yourself, and giving yourself a break. If your depression lasts for more than 4 weeks, contact your physician to explore other alternatives.

You can also treat yourself to natural healing support by using essential oil blends. Not only will the natural chemicals from the plants help equalize your hormonal levels, but their soothing scents can also help lift your spirits.

Essential Oil Blends

Essential oils that are helpful in balancing hormones are:

- Chamomile, Geranium, Patchouli, and Ylang Ylang for weepiness

- Clary Sage, Cypress, Grapefruit, and Rosemary for lethargic depression

- Cedarwood, Sandalwood, and Vetiver for emotional release

- Bergamot, Chamomile, Cypress, Marjoram, and Rosemary for emotional exhaustion

Refer to the "Essential Oil Chart" for contraindications, warnings, or cautions about using essential oils.

Refer to the "Emotional Support" chapter to learn more about scent therapy. In addition to offering support to counteract the blues, the Baby Blues Soother is great to use in the evening to relax and feel at peace. *This blend has a nice combination of a hormonal regulator and a mild sedative. I used this after my 2:00 feeding to get right back to sleep.*

Baby Blues Soother

10 drops Cedarwood

5 drops Geranium

8 drops Sandalwood

5 drops Vetiver

> When you want to create a blend that you can smell and that absorbs into the skin, you can make a body oil or a body splash.
>
> Add all of the essential oils to 2 tablespoons of carrier oil (any oil listed in the "Carrier Oils" chapter). Shake well and dab on your pulse points and at the base of your neck 4 to 6 times daily for the first week. If you notice an improvement, you can reduce the applications to 2 to 3 times daily until your depression subsides.
>
> To make a body splash, add all of the essential oils to 8 ounces of water in a spray bottle. Spritz (3 – 5 squirts) your upper body (upper chest and neck area) 4 to 6 times daily for the first week. If you notice an improvement, you can reduce the applications to 2 to 3 times daily until your depression subsides.

Note: If you do not notice improvement at the end of the first week, continue to use the blend 4 to 6 times daily for up to 6 weeks. Progress with emotional concerns varies by individual.

You may want to continue to use the blend once daily simply to avoid the recurrence of depression.

When you use the Postpartum Depression Relief blend, you feel uplifted, confident, and certain but without an excessive or manic feeling. Use this blend during the day to stay focused and balanced.

Postpartum Depression Relief

10 drops Bergamot

5 drops Clary Sage

5 drops Geranium

8 drops Grapefruit

When you want to create a blend that you can smell and that absorbs into the skin, you can make a body oil or a body splash.

Add all of the essential oils to 2 tablespoons of carrier oil (any oil listed in the "Carrier Oils" chapter). Shake well and dab on your pulse points and at the base of your neck 4 to 6 times daily for the first week. If you notice an improvement, you can reduce the applications to 2 to 3 times daily until your depression subsides.

To make a body splash, add all of the essential oils to 8 ounces of water in a spray bottle. Spritz (3 – 5 squirts) your upper body (upper chest and neck area) 4 to 6 times daily for the first week. If you notice an improvement, you can reduce the applications to 2 to 3 times daily until your depression subsides.

Note: If you do not notice improvement at the end of the first week, continue to use the blend 4 to 6 times daily for up to 6 weeks. Progress with emotional concerns varies by individual.

You may want to continue to use the blend once daily simply to avoid the recurrence of depression.

Stress

"Peace and friendship with all mankind is our wisest policy, and I wish we may be permitted to pursue it."

Thomas Jefferson

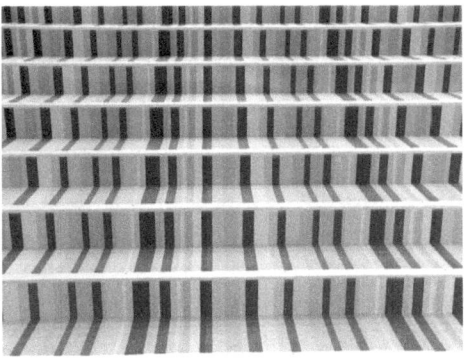

In the frantic world of today that we live in, it feels that we are not permitted to pursue peace and friendship. The result is often stress. Stop for just a moment, close your eyes, take some deep breaths, and imagine a peaceful place. I know you feel better. But I also know you can't spend all day with your eyes closed, so read on and let essential oils help.

I could write an entire book about stress — many people have. The reason I provide a brief description of the characteristics of an ailment is to give you confidence that the aromatherapy blends suggested are based on my understanding of the ailment. Here's what I consider when I formulate blends for stress. Stress is one way the body defends itself. However, too much stress can lead to physical concerns such as back pain, constipation or diarrhea, fatigue, headaches, high blood pressure, insomnia, weight gain or loss, and more. Before that happens you need to intervene.

Stress can be caused by literally anything because what may be stressful to one person may not be to another. Common causes of stress include getting laid off from your job, your child leaving or returning home, the death of your spouse, divorce or marriage, an illness, an injury, a job promotion, money problems, moving, or having a baby.

In addition to basic healthy living: eating a balanced diet, getting plenty of sleep, exercising, and avoiding caffeine and tobacco; there are other strategies that may help you deal with stress. Identify the things that cause you stress; take control of the things you can influence; and let the other things go. Ask yourself what you are worried about. If you can do something about it – do it. If you can't do anything about it – don't worry about it. Easier said than done, I know, but oh so necessary.

As you will see with these essential oil blends, you can have safe and effective natural support all day long. But do notice that I also suggest a nice soothing bath. Just taking time for yourself on a daily basis will have a tremendous positive influence on your reaction to stress. Remember, by selecting certain letters from the word stress, you can spell rest.

Essential Oil Blends

Essential oils that are effective in supporting your emotional well being are: Geranium, Lavender, and Ylang Ylang for tiredness and irritability; Cedarwood and Myrrh to release tension; Chamomile, Clary Sage, Geranium, Lavender, and Sandalwood for anxiety, fear, and despair; and Bergamot, Frankincense, Lemon, Marjoram,

Nutmeg, and Vetiver for general symptoms of stress. Refer to the "Essential Oil Chart" for contraindications, warnings, or cautions about using essential oils.

Get the most out of your bath time by adding the Take Me Away blend to your bath.

It would almost seem that if you could find 20 minutes each day to take a bath, you wouldn't need additional support to relieve stress.

Take Me Away From Stress

4 drops Bergamot

2 drops Clary Sage

4 drops Lavender

> Mix all oils in a nice warm bath. Close the door, slide in, and relax for 20 minutes.

> On the days that you can't enjoy a bath, try this instead: after your shower, apply a few drops of this blend to your wet facecloth and gently rub all over your body.

If you did get a bath, and have someone available to spoil you, use the Massage Away Stress blend to do just that.

Massage Away Stress

4 drops Cedar

1 drop Myrrh

3 drops Sandalwood

> Mix all oils in one ounce of carrier oil. Rub this all over your skin.

When you need stress relieving assistance outside of the bath (and isn't that usually where we need it?), you can mix up the Stress Reduction blend and put all of the essential oils in a cup of water in a spray bottle. Spritz your body, your office, or your home to get daytime stress relief.

Note: Do NOT spray this blend in your car as some of the essential oils have a mild sedative effect.

Stress Reduction

10 drops Chamomile

5 drops Geranium

10 drops Lavender

5 drops Lemon

> Mix oils together. Put 8 drops of the blend into a soothing bath or sauna. The same blend, diluted in 2 tablespoons of carrier oil, applied to the temples, back of the neck, across the forehead, and behind the ears is a wonderful relief for stress-induced headaches.

Family Care

Can you use essential oils on all members of the family, including pets?

The short answer to this question is yes. Many of the recipes in *Aromatherapy Answers* are formulated for particular age groups. Following the instructions carefully will make sure you are making safe and effective blends for all members of the family. To be more specific, there are only a limited number of essential oils that are safe to use for children under the age of three. Be sure you look for recipes that indicate that you can use the blend on small children. Also, for the very elderly who typically have more fragile constitutions and skin, you can reduce the "adult" formulas by 25% so that these recipes are safe and will still be effective. For pets, you reduce many blends by almost 90% because pets are smaller than humans (in most cases), and are extremely receptive to the benefits of essential oils.

The remainder of this section deals with:

- Bronchitis
- Colds
- Congestion
- Constipation
- Coughs
- Dandruff
- Earaches
- Flu Fighters
- Headaches
- Immune System

- Indigestion
- Sinus

Bronchitis

"We shall breathe the air again"

George Frederick Root

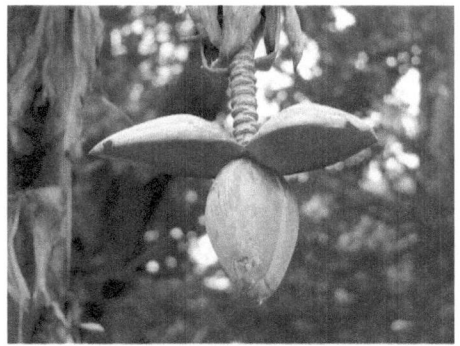

With bronchitis, breathing the air again seems impossible. You know you've got it before you even go to the doctor's office. In fact, knowing you had it made you make that appointment. You've had it before; perhaps it is your body's favorite winter malady. What can start out as a simple (but annoying) head cold can turn into bronchitis. Wouldn't it be great to head it off at the pass? Or failing that, make the journey through somewhat easier? Then read on.

Bronchitis is an inflammation of the bronchial tubes, or bronchi (the air passages that extend from the windpipe into the lungs). A virus, bacterial infection, smoking, or the inhalation of chemical pollutants or dust can cause the inflammation. When the cells of the bronchial-lining tissue are irritated, the air passages become clogged, irritation increases, and mucus develops, and causes the characteristic cough of bronchitis. Brief bouts of acute bronchitis often evolve from a cold or the flu. Acute bronchitis usually lasts about 10 days.

The most effective way to deal with acute bronchitis is to get plenty of rest, stay warm, and drink lots of fluid. Do not use a cough suppressant, as you want to get rid of the congestive mucus. Your doctor may recommend an expectorant to help loosen the mucus. Consult your doctor if the sputum (the mucus mixed with saliva) produced by the coughing is greenish-yellow and thick rather than gray and watery, or if your fever rises or chest pains become severe.

Chronic bronchitis is defined as excessive mucus secretion in the bronchi with a chronic or recurrent mucus-producing cough that lasts three or more months and recurs year after year. Chronic bronchitis may result from a series of attacks of acute bronchitis, or it may evolve gradually from heavy smoking or the inhalation of air contaminated with other pollutants in the environment.

To loosen up mucus, try hot or spicy foods. Avoid dairy products. Many soups can offer comfort. Hot and Sour soup will probably make your nose run, but that lets you know it is thinning mucus. Other foods you probably don't think of as sickbed food are helpful, too: salsa, horseradish, and wasabi, to name a few.

In addition to spicy food, hot drinks are helpful for thinning mucus and will soothe your throat as well. Keeping hydrated is always a good idea when you don't feel well. Drink plenty of hot tea. Ginger tea is particularly helpful because the ginger helps clear congestion.

Speak to your doctor about vitamins and supplements that can be helpful, such as vitamin C, Golden Seal, Echinacea, and zinc.

Echinacea and zinc should only be taken for a limited time (up to seven days).

Essential Oil Blends

The best essential oils for upper respiratory issues are Cedarwood, Clove, Cypress, Eucalyptus, Ginger, Lavender, Lemon, Peppermint, Rosemary, Tea Tree, and Thyme. Refer to the "Essential Oil Chart" for contraindications, warnings, or cautions about using essential oils.

The following aromatherapy blends can be used as inhalants or as massage blends. Let your personal preference guide you. With the Teen and Adult Bronchitis Basher, you can attack the bronchitis from every angle. This is an extremely potent blend when used as directed.

Teen and Adult Bronchitis Basher

12 drops Clove

12 drops Cypress

16 drops Eucalyptus

8 drops Lemon

8 drops Peppermint

8 drops Rosemary

8 drops Thyme

Mix all the essential oils together in a dark glass container. For the first 3 days, run a cool mist vaporizer. Put 12 drops of the combined essential oil blend in the vaporizer (see information about vaporizers in the "Introduction" chapter). You can also put 12 drops in a pot of boiling water, REMOVE from the heat, and breathe in the scented steam. Use hot steam on a limited basis only.

You can also add 32 drops of the essential oil blend to 2 ounces of base lotion or 2 tablespoons of carrier oil (any oil listed in the "Carrier Oils" chapter). Apply a small amount of the blend to your chest, back, neck, and behind your ears. Apply the blend at least 4 to 6 times a day until your symptoms subside. You can expect relief within 3 – 5 days.

Note: If you are well enough to get out of bed for work, school, etc., apply the blend to the bottom of your feet before you start the day so you can pump the essential oils into your bloodstream when you walk.

Leave the remaining essential oil blend in the brown bottle, and take it with you. Inhale the blend several times during the day for additional relief. You can either inhale it straight from the bottle or put a few drops on a tissue.

With so many essential oils that have the natural chemical properties to treat bronchitis, I looked for a combination of oils that would work against the bronchitis, but also provide some emotional support during a time when you are feeling downright lousy.

The Bronchitis Blaster takes care of the bronchitis and also makes you feel like Mom is there with you pouring on the sympathy and tender loving care. What could be better?

Bronchitis Blaster

8 drops Cinnamon

8 drops Clove

16 drops Eucalyptus

8 drops Ginger

8 drops Nutmeg

16 drops Thyme

Mix all the essential oils together in a dark glass container. For the first 3 days, run a cool mist vaporizer. Put 10 drops of the combined essential oil blend in the vaporizer (see information about vaporizers in the "Introduction" chapter). You can also put 10 drops in a pot of boiling water, REMOVE from the heat, and breathe in the scented steam. Use hot steam on a limited basis only.

You can also add 32 drops of the essential oil blend to 2 ounces of base lotion or 2 tablespoons of carrier oil (any oil listed in the "Carrier Oils" chapter). Apply a small amount of the blend to your chest, back, neck, and behind your ears. Apply the blend at least 4 to 6 times a day until your symptoms subside. You can expect relief within 3 – 5 days.

Note: If you are well enough to get out of bed for work, school, etc., apply the blend to the bottom of your feet before you start the day so you can pump the essential oils into your bloodstream when you walk.

Leave the remaining essential oil blend in the brown bottle, and take it with you. Inhale the blend several times during the day for additional relief. You can either inhale it straight from the bottle or put a few drops on a tissue.

The Respiratory Ailments blend is safe enough to use on children ages three years and older. For children under three years, delete the Rosemary oil from the blend.

Respiratory Ailments Remedy

10 drops Eucalyptus

10 drops Lavender

10 drops Rosemary

10 drops Tea Tree

>Mix all oils together. Use your blend in any of the following ways:

>Use 10 drops in a cool-mist vaporizer (see information about vaporizers in the "Introduction" chapter).

>Put 2 drops on a cotton ball and tuck inside the child's pillow.

>Use 1 drop in a tub of warm water for a pleasant bath.

Common Colds

"But Mr. Jeremy liked getting his feet wet; nobody ever scolded him, and he never caught a cold."

Beatrix Potter

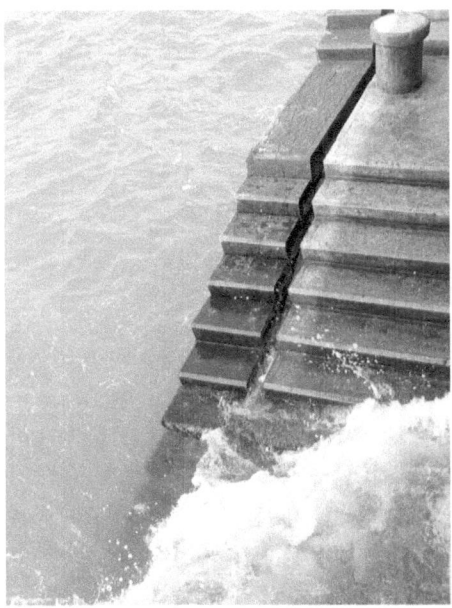

Out of the blue you sneeze — and you know you are catching a cold. Whether you got too tired and exposed to many germs, or your child has a classroom full of sneezing classmates, you now have a cold. Guess what? Now you will have it for 7 days or more depending on how you treat it. Aromatherapy can help you keep your environment more antiseptic to help you avoid colds, and it can help keep your loved ones from catching your cold. And, if you get a cold – in spite of all your precautions — aromatherapy can help you deal with the symptoms and feel better faster.

Viruses cause colds; in fact, there are over 100 different viruses that can cause the common cold. People of all ages, gender, and overall health get colds. A cold often starts with fatigue, sneezing, coughing, and a runny nose. You may also run a low-grade fever, have muscle aches, a scratchy or sore throat, watery eyes, and a headache.

If you have a cold, there are things you can do to make yourself feel better. Stay home and rest, especially while you have a fever. Stop smoking and avoid secondhand smoke. Drink plenty of fluids like water, fruit juices, herbal teas, and clear soups. Avoid alcohol. Gargle with warm salt water a few times a day to relieve a sore throat. Throat sprays or lozenges may also help relieve the pain. Use salt water (saline) nose drops to help loosen mucus and moisten the tender skin in your nose.

You should contact your doctor if your cold lasts more than 10 days, if you have a high fever, shortness of breath, wheezing, or a cough that just won't go away.

You can also try that age-old remedy, chicken soup (lovingly referred to as Jewish penicillin), which is soothing and helps your nose run. Now that may not be an attractive thought, but anything that get that mucus moving is helpful in getting you to feel better faster. Interestingly enough, hot spices and garlic also have therapeutic value and will give that soup more flavor (no offense Grandma) — something you and your stuffed up nose might really appreciate.

And don't forget the vitamin C. You can find it in orange juice and warm drinks, as well as in supplements.

Speak to your doctor about vitamins and supplements that can be helpful, such as Golden Seal, Colloidal Silver, Echinacea, and Zinc. Echinacea and Zinc should only be taken for a limited time (up to seven days).

Essential Oil Blends

The best essential oils for colds are Eucalyptus, Lavender, Pine, and Spruce. Refer to the "Essential Oil Chart" for contraindications, warnings, or cautions about using essential oils.

You will want to use these blends to ease your breathing, help clear mucus, and keep the environment fresh and clean smelling. The Child and Youngster Cold Relief blend contains essential oils that are safe enough to use on children as young as three years old. You can also use this blend for younger children, but ONLY in a cool-mist vaporizer or diffuser.

Child and Youngster Cold Relief

20 drops Eucalyptus

20 drops Lavender

20 drops Tea Tree

> Mix all oils together. Use in any or all of the following ways:
>
> Put 15 drops in a cool-mist vaporizer at bedtime (see information about vaporizers in the "Introduction" chapter). In the morning, if the cold still stifles your child's breathing, clean the vaporizer and add 3 drops to clean water.
>
> For heavy congestion during the night, put 2 drops on a piece of cotton and tuck it inside your resting child's pillowcase.
>
> Put 2 drops in a bath. Not only will the steam help clear out nasal passages, but also the calming properties of this blend will help your child rest.
>
> Add 15 drops to 2 teaspoons of carrier oil, and massage your child's lung area (chest and back).

Teens and adults can use essential oils that have a bit more punch. The Teen and Adult Cold Relief blend is not only very effective in treating the symptoms of common colds, but also has a wonderful invigorating fragrance.

When I have a head cold, the Teen and Adult Cold Relief blend is very comforting when mixed into a carrier oil and massaged on my sinus areas. It works best for bedtime when my eyes will be closed (the essential oils are pretty potent) and I can feel the warm sensation helping to loosen up all that is clogging my head.

Teen and Adult Cold Relief

8 drops Eucalyptus

12 drops Geranium

8 drops Peppermint

12 drops Rosemary

> Mix all oils together. Use in any or all of the following ways:
>
> Put 15 drops in a cool-mist vaporizer at bedtime (see information about vaporizers in the "Introduction" chapter). Children are not the only people to benefit from steam inhalation.
>
> Put 2 drops on a tissue and carry with you for a brief blast of relief.
>
> Put 4 drops in a bath. Not only will the steam help clear out nasal passages, but also the calming properties of this blend will help you rest.
>
> Add 15 drops to 2 tablespoons of vegetable oil, and massage the lung area (chest and back), neck, around the ears, forehead, nose, and cheekbones.

As soon as I turn on the heat for the winter season, I also turn on the cool-mist vaporizer and use the Vaporizer Blend (see information about vaporizers in the "Introduction" chapter). For just pennies a day, I can avoid the miseries associated with being sick – spending too much time at the doctor's office, spending too much money on medications, spending too much time away from my family; it's all just too much. See how powerful this blend is in keeping you healthy through cold and flu season.

Vaporizer Blend for the Entire Family

6 drops Eucalyptus

4 drops Lavender

2 drop Peppermint

4 drops Rosemary

> Mix the oils together. Add to a full cool-mist vaporizer. Add 15 to 30 drops of the blend to the water in your vaporizer. Day 1 – fill vaporizer and put in 15 drops of oils. Day 2 – just refill the water to the top (that is if the water reduces about 1/3 of the way). Day 3 – just refill the water to the top (that is if the water reduces about 1/3 of the way). Day 4 – empty vaporizer, clean it out, and start at Day 1 again.

Congestion

"Happy the man whose wish and care; a few paternal acres bound,
Content to breathe his native air in his own ground."

Alexander Pope

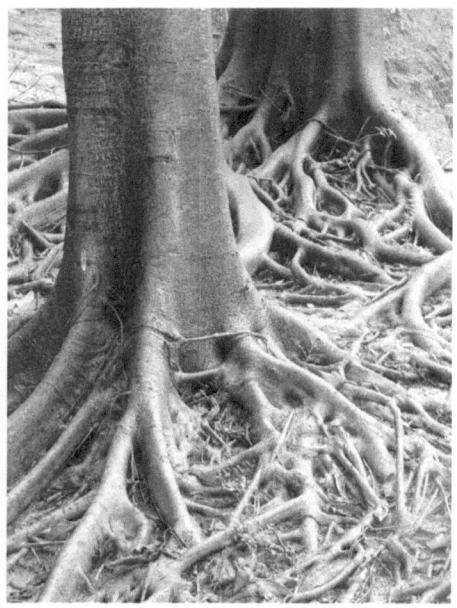

Your breathing is labored. Your nose feels like each molecule of air has to fight its way up. You are congested and every breathing passage feels swollen. Use aromatherapy to help open passages and breath more freely.

Congestion is caused by the inflammation of the mucus membrane in the bronchial tubes. The inflammation is triggered by bacteria, viruses, and other environmental and chemical agents such as dust and fumes. You know you have congestion because of the incessant coughing, back and chest pain, and difficulty breathing.

To help ease the congestion, drink plenty of fluids to break up the mucus and make it easier to cough up. Interestingly enough, caffeine, especially hot and steamy coffee, helps to open your air passages. You can also use a cool-mist vaporizer to break up mucus. And, most importantly, cough to get rid of the mucus. You don't want to take a cough suppressant because you are trying to expel the mucus from your lungs.

If your symptoms are significant or if mild symptoms persist for more than 5 days, go to the doctor to explore treatment options. Contact a doctor immediately if you have a high fever or you are wheezing, having trouble breathing, or coughing up green or brown phlegm.

If you feel like eating, try hot and spicy food, which will help break up the mucus. Probably the first symptom of thinning mucus will be a runny nose. Grab that box of tissues and rejoice; things are starting to move on out!

Essential Oil Blends

The best essential oils for congestion are Clove, Eucalyptus, Frankincense, Lemon, Oregano, Peppermint, Sage, Tea Tree, and Thyme. Refer to the "Essential Oil Chart" for contraindications, warnings, or cautions about using essential oils.

The following aromatherapy blends can be used as either inhalants or massage blends. Let your personal preference guide you. The Respiratory Ailments Remedy has helped hundreds of people who enjoyed my first aromatherapy book.

Respiratory Ailments Remedy

10 drops Eucalyptus

10 drops Lavender

10 drops Rosemary

10 drops Tea Tree

> Mix all the oils together in a dark glass container. Use this blend in any of the following ways:
>
> 10 drops in a diffuser during the day. After one use, refresh the water and add 3 drops of the blend for use at night.
>
> Use 1 drop in a tub of warm water for a pleasant bath.
>
> Put 2 drops on a cotton ball and tuck inside your pillow.

Call it psychological, but clients frequently prefer the Congestion Relief blend during the fall and winter months. I don't know if the scent of Clove makes you think that something is baking or if the uplifting properties of Lemon promise warmer days. It could be a little of both.

Congestion Relief

10 drops Clove

16 drops Eucalyptus

20 drops Lemon

16 drops Tea Tree

16 drops Thyme

Mix all the oils together in a dark glass container. For the first 3 days, run a cool mist vaporizer (see information about vaporizers in the "Introduction" chapter). Put 10 drops of the combined essential oil blend in the vaporizer.

Then, add 28 drops of the essential oil blend to 2 ounces of lotion or 2 tablespoons of carrier oil (any oil listed in the "Carrier Oils" chapter). Apply a small amount of the blend to your chest, back, neck, and behind your ears. Apply the blend at least 4 to 6 times a day until your symptoms subside. You can expect relief within 3 – 5 days.

Note: If you are well enough to get out of bed for work, school, etc., apply the blend to the bottom of your feet before you start the day so you can pump the essential oils into your bloodstream when you walk.

Leave the remaining essential oil blend in the brown bottle, and take it with you. Inhale the blend several times during the day for additional relief. You can either inhale it straight from the bottle or put a few drops on a tissue.

Congestion Soother not only offers relief from upper respiratory problems, but also contains essential oils that support your mental and emotional health during your time of illness.

Congestion Soother

10 drops Cinnamon

16 drops Eucalyptus

8 drops Frankincense

8 drops Peppermint

16 drops Rosemary

Mix all the oils together in a dark glass container. For the first 3 days, run a cool mist vaporizer (see information about vaporizers in the "Introduction" chapter). Put 10 drops of the combined essential oil blend in the vaporizer.

You can also add 28 drops of the essential oil blend to 2 ounces of lotion or 2 tablespoons of carrier oil (any oil listed in the "Carrier Oils" chapter). Apply a small amount of the blend to your chest, back, neck, and behind your ears. Apply the blend at least 4 to 6 times a day until your symptoms subside. You can expect relief within 3 – 5 days.

Note: If you are well enough to get out of bed for work, school, etc., apply the blend to the bottom of your feet before you start the day so you can pump the essential oils into your bloodstream when you walk.

Leave the remaining essential oil blend in the brown bottle, and take it with you. Inhale the blend several times during the day for additional relief. You can either inhale it straight from the bottle or put a few drops on a tissue.

Note: Take care with the cinnamon essential oil. If it touches your skin wash it off with soap and warm water. While cinnamon smells delicious, if left on skin it can cause a burning sensation that can become quite uncomfortable.

Constipation

"Don't squat with your spurs on."

Will Rogers

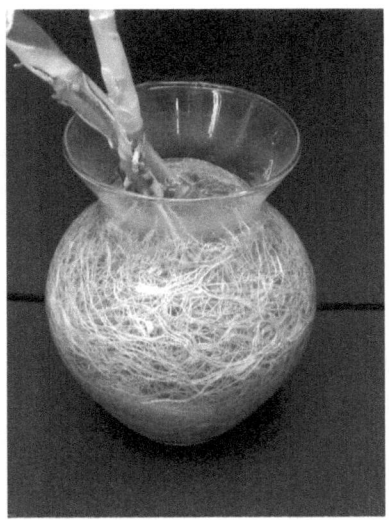

There is nothing funny about constipation, but when I saw this quote I just had to share it with you, because people who suffer with constipation are willing to try just about anything.

The most common gastrointestinal disorder in the United States, constipation is the condition of infrequent (usually fewer than three times a week) bowel movements of dry and hardened feces. Other symptoms include feeling bloated, uncomfortable, and sluggish. In most cases, constipation is temporary and not serious.

Those suffering from constipation most often are women, children, and adults aged 65 and over. Pregnant women often complain of constipation. It is a common problem following childbirth or surgery.

The causes of constipation are: poor diet (not enough fiber and liquids), lack of exercise, certain medications, stress, and other changes such as pregnancy, aging, and travel.

The National Digestive Diseases Information Clearinghouse (NDDIC) offers the following advice to help relieve symptoms of and prevent constipation:

- Eat a well-balanced, high-fiber diet that includes beans, bran, whole grains, fresh fruits, and vegetables.

- Drink plenty of liquids, including prune juice and even coffee.

- Exercise regularly.

- Set aside time after breakfast or dinner for undisturbed visits to the toilet.

- Do not ignore the urge to have a bowel movement.

- Understand that normal bowel habits vary.

- Whenever a significant or prolonged change in bowel habits occurs, check with your doctor.

Essential Oil Blends

Essential oils that assist in aiding digestion are Black Pepper, Cinnamon, Fennel, Ginger, Nutmeg, Orange, Palma Rosa, Peppermint, and Tangerine. Chamomile, Marjoram, Patchouli, and Yarrow are soothing to the digestive tract. Refer to the "Essential

Oil Chart" for contraindications, warnings, or cautions about using essential oils.

I have found a helpful, yet quick and easy, way to get my system going most days is to drink a mug full of warm (almost tea temperature) water with one teaspoon of lemon juice in it as soon as I get up. Then I brush my teeth because the lemon juice makes them feel funny. The scientific reason for this is that lemon juice promotes peristalsis (muscular contractions) in the colon.

The Constipation Relief blend is great for adults who suffer from frequent constipation. I would suggest that you also make the Muesli recipe at the end of this section. Use both of these treatments to see if you can regulate your bowel movements.

Constipation Relief

6 drops Fennel

6 drops Ginger

4 drops Peppermint

> Add all essential oils to 2 ounces of base lotion or 2 tablespoons of carrier oil (any oil listed in the "Carrier Oils" chapter). **Gently** apply a small amount of the blend to the abdomen and to the lower back around the kidney area in soft, circular motions. Apply the blend 4 to 6 times a day until you have comfortable bowel movements. You can expect relief within 7 – 10 days.

The Constipation Soother blend is more appropriate for children, young adults, and for people who only suffer constipation occasionally. If you fit into this category, you may also want to keep a record of what your life was about just before the constipation occurred. Write down what was going on; what you ate and drank, your sleeping habits, etc. You might find a trigger that brought about the constipation. And, with constipation, you are better off avoiding it all together.

Constipation Soother

4 drops Chamomile

6 drops Patchouli

6 drops Tangerine

> Add all essential oils to 2 ounces of base lotion or 2 tablespoons of carrier oil (any oil listed in the "Carrier Oils" chapter). **Gently** apply a small amount of the blend to the lower back around the kidney area in soft, circular motions. Apply the blend 4 to 6 times a day until you have comfortable bowel movements. You can expect relief within 7 – 10 days.

This natural cereal tastes great, works wonderfully, and is easy to make.

Bircher Muesli

1 tablespoon oats

3 tablespoons water or apple juice

1 tablespoon evaporated milk or soya milk

1 tablespoon grated or whole nuts

1 large grated apple with the peel

1 drop Lemon

> Soak the oats overnight in the apple juice or water, in the refrigerator. Before breakfast, grate the apple and add to the rest of the ingredients.

When I was pregnant, I made up about one week's worth of the oats, juice, and milk every Sunday. Then each day I would only have to grate the apple and add the nuts. Be sure to keep it refrigerated.

This recipe was excerpted from the *Complete Book of Essential Oils and Aromatherapy* by Valerie Ann Worwood.

Coughs

"Love, and a cough, cannot be hid."

George Herbert

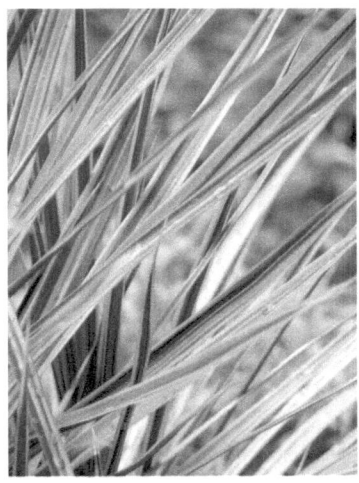

You wonder what's worse: that little dry tickle cough that seems to erupt from you in the middle of a meeting or phone call, or that heavy cough that means business. Some coughs seem so deeply rooted that you actually feel pain in your chest while coughing.

There are two basic types of cough: chesty and dry. If you have mucus or phlegm, you have a chesty cough. No mucus or phlegm? You have a dry cough.

When you have a chesty cough, coughing is beneficial because it helps move the mucus out of your chest. You have heard about a productive cough (I always thought that was a joke) but that means a cough that is moving the mucus out of your chest. With a dry cough, coughing has no benefit and is just a bother.

Some of the best ways to relieve symptoms of coughs are tried and true folk remedies. Inhaling steam (via a hot bath or shower) helps to break up chest congestion and soothes the chest. You can also use a cool mist vaporizer. If you choose an over-the-counter cough syrup, be sure you choose the cough solution that meets your specific needs. With a dry cough, you want to stop the urge to cough. With a chesty cough you want to aid your natural coughing to get rid of the phlegm.

Essential Oil Blends

The best essential oils for coughs are Bergamot, Chamomile, Cypress, Eucalyptus, Frankincense, Ginger, Lemon, Tea Tree, and Thyme. Refer to the "Essential Oil Chart" for contraindications, warnings, or cautions about using essential oils.

When I was a little girl I had chronic coughs. I remember my mother holding me in her arms, rocking me back and forth, as she sat on the side of the bathtub. With hot steaming water filling the small room, she would hold me and sing to me until I settled down. I didn't like being sick, but I loved those special close times with my mom.

You can use these blends to ease your breathing, keep your mucus clear, and keep the environment fresh and clean smelling. When you want a natural expectorant to assist your body, use the Cough Relief blend. Most people use this blend during the day when they can tolerate a productive cough.

Cough Relief

15 drops Eucalyptus

15 drops Lavender

15 drops Tea Tree

15 drops Thyme

> Mix all the oils together in a dark glass container. Use this blend in either of these ways:
>
> For the first 3 days, run a cool mist vaporizer (see information about vaporizers in the "Introduction" chapter). Put 10 drops of the combined essential oil blend in the vaporizer.
>
> You can also add 28 drops of the essential oil blend to 2 ounces of base lotion or 2 tablespoons of carrier oil (any oil listed in the "Carrier Oils" chapter). Apply a small amount of the blend to your chest, back, neck, and behind your ears. Apply the blend at least 4 to 6 times a day until your symptoms subside. You can expect relief within 3 – 5 days.

Note: If you are well enough to get out of bed for work, school, etc., apply the blend to the bottom of your feet before you start the day so you can pump the essential oils into your bloodstream when you walk.

> Leave the remaining essential oil blend in the brown bottle, and take it with you. Inhale the blend several times during the day for additional relief. You can either inhale it straight from the bottle or put a few drops on a tissue.

When you are tired and need a good night's sleep, use the Cough Soother. Even though you have the natural expectorant in Eucalyptus, you also have some gentle yet effective sedatives in Chamomile and Lavender.

Cough Soother

10 drops Chamomile

10 drops Eucalyptus

10 drops Lavender

10 drops Rosemary

10 drops Tea Tree

Mix all oils together. Use this blend in either of these ways:

Use 3 drops in a diffuser during the day. After one use, refresh the water and add 3 drops of the blend for use at night.

Mix between 10 and 20 drops of the blend in 2 tablespoons carrier oil to massage your chest and back (lung area) three times a day.

Dandruff

"They crowned him long ago ... with a diadem of snow"

Lord Byron

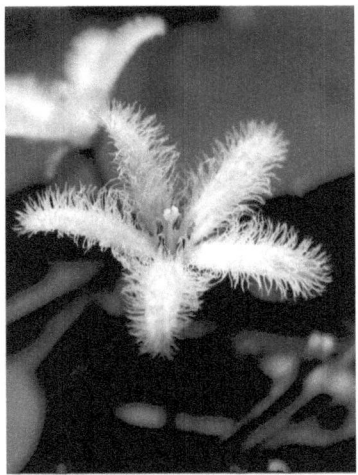

You have an interview and are wearing your good navy blazer. Your scalp itches a bit. You scratch — to your horror you notice white flakes on your shoulder! There's a good chance you have dandruff; nothing private about it either. Even if you refrain from scratching, the flakes of dead skin released by your scalp will be on your shoulders within the hour for the world to see. The next time you have snow on your crown, be sure that it's not dandruff.

Dandruff is seborrheic dermatitis, an inflammation of the scalp caused by a common, yeast-like organism found on the scalp and other parts of human skin. While many natural fungi do not have harmful effects, certain stressors, such as climate, stress, and hormonal changes can trigger the fungus to grow. Your skin becomes more irritated and the rate at which skin cells shed increases. That is what gives the visible appearance of dandruff.

The symptoms of dandruff can increase during times of poor nutrition, stress, or infection. Excessive use of hair products and hair dryers can cause some symptoms of dandruff. But true dandruff itches as well. Because dandruff is an inflammation, vitamin C may be helpful because of its anti-inflammatory properties.

Essential Oil Blends

The best essential oils for dandruff are Cedarwood, Lavender, Lemon, Patchouli, Peppermint, Rosemary, Sage, Tea Tree, and Thyme. Refer to the "Essential Oil Chart" for contraindications, warnings, or cautions about using essential oils.

While there are a lot of harsh dandruff treatments available commercially, you can be tender and loving to your hair and get rid of that dandruff too.

As you can see from the list of oils that are recommended for dandruff, you have many options. The blends offered here have worked most effectively for my clients.

Dandruff Shampoo for Teens and Adults

4 drops Cedarwood

6 drops Lavender

4 drops Rosemary

8 drops Tea Tree

> Mix all essential oils and add the oils to 4 ounces of baby shampoo. Wash your hair as usual. After three weeks if you feel you are getting the moisturizing relief that you want, then this is the right blend for you!
>
> For additional moisturizing, you can add 15 drops of additional moisturizing oils, such as Evening Primrose, Borage Seed, or Vitamin E. Pin prick the gel caps and squeeze the contents into the shampoo.

Warning: Some of the properties of Cedarwood may have abortive effects and thus Cedarwood should not be used in any form during pregnancy.

Sometimes the hormonal fluctuation of pregnancy brings about dandruff for women who have never suffered with it before. This blend is safe enough for you to use during those wonderful months or pregnancy.

Dandruff Shampoo for Children and Pregnant Women

6 drops Carrot

4 drops Eucalyptus

8 drops Lavender

4 drops Lemon

> Mix all essential oils and add the oils to 4 ounces of the baby shampoo. Wash your hair as usual. After three weeks if you feel you are getting the moisturizing relief that you want, then this is the right blend for you!

> For additional moisturizing, you can add 15 drops of additional moisturizing oils, such as Evening Primrose, Borage Seed, or Vitamin E. Pin prick the gel caps and squeeze the contents into the shampoo.

The Hair Rinse for Dandruff gives you another alternative to help relieve dandruff. We suggest that you use this rinse every few months to help keep the natural organisms in your body balanced. Even if you don't have dandruff, it's a nice preventive treatment.

Hair Rinse for Dandruff

5 drops Eucalyptus

10 drops Rosemary

5 drops Tea Tree

> Mix all of the essential oils in either 2 Tablespoons cider vinegar (for brunettes) or 2 Tablespoons lemon juice (for blonds). Pour this mixture in one cup of water. After washing your hair with a mild shampoo, pour the rinse over your head, taking care to keep it out of your eyes. Rinse with warm water.

For a bit of pampering to your head, try the warm oil treatments that follow. The first blend is specifically formulated to treat dandruff.

Scalp Oil Treatment for Dandruff

4 drops Cedarwood

8 drops Lavender

2 drops Lemon

4 drops Rosemary

4 drops Tea Tree

> Mix all oils together in 2 tablespoons of olive oil. Use the entire blend to massage on your scalp thoroughly. Wrap your head with a hot towel or plastic wrap and relax for one hour. Shampoo and rinse. You may have to shampoo twice to remove all the olive oil.

Note: To make a towel hot, wet it with hot water and wring it out or microwave it.

Warning: Some of the properties of Cedarwood may have abortive effects and thus Cedarwood should not be used in any form during pregnancy.

This is the scalp treatment of choice for me. I color treat my hair, swim about 5 times a week, and, let's see what other things do I do that my hair hates? Oh yes, wear my hair stuffed in a cap when I am coaching or gardening. This seems to suffocate my scalp. So, as you can imagine, I occasionally have itchy scalp and some minor flakes. Just thinking about how wonderful I feel when I use this blend, you are going to have to excuse me; I'm going to take advantage of it right now. I wonder how dreamy and relaxed the next section of the book is going to sound.

Warm Oil Treatment for Damaged Hair

2 drops Cedarwood

6 drops Clary Sage

2 drops Geranium

2 drops Lavender

6 drops Rosemary

Mix all oils together in 2 tablespoons of olive oil. You can use this blend in one of two ways:

Massage blend on hair and scalp. Make sure you reach those split ends. Wrap your head with a hot towel or plastic wrap and relax for one hour. Shampoo and rinse; be sure to rinse well to remove the olive oil.

Note: To make a towel hot, wet it with hot water and wring it out or microwave it.

Add a few drops of this blend to a mild shampoo and use on a regular basis when you wash your hair.

Warning: Some of the properties of Cedarwood may have abortive effects and thus Cedarwood should not be used in any form during pregnancy.

Earaches

"Blessed is the man, who having nothing to say, abstains from giving wordy evidence of the fact."

George Eliot

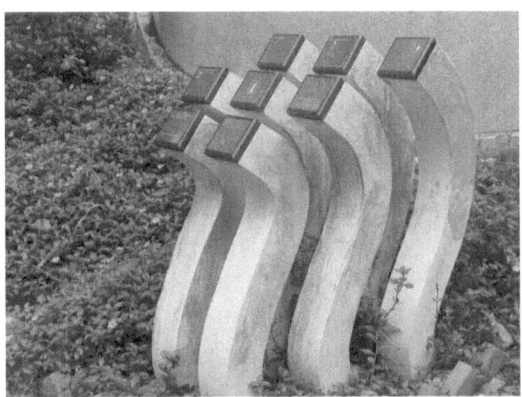

When we are in the company of people who do not take this great author's advice, we just want to plug our ears and not listen. However, if you have an earache, you would rather listen to some long-winded speech, than suffer the pain and discomfort of your earache. And, doesn't it seem that your earache is worse at night, so you not only suffer from the pain, but also from lack of sleep?

Nothing breaks a mother's heart more than when her child is in pain. Unfortunately, about 75% of all children (more boys than girls) will have at least one earache before they are three years old. Earaches commonly occur when the Eustachian tube becomes blocked. This prevents fluid from draining out of the tube. This blockage can occur because of allergies, a cold, or other infection. Acute ear infections usually clear up within 1 or 2 weeks. The most common symptoms of an acute ear infection are ear pain (which may be sudden and severe) and fever.

There are several things you can do to help your child avoid getting an earache. Keep them away from cigarette smoke, out of germy environments, and don't let them take a bottle to bed.

Once your child has an ear infection, you should see your doctor. In addition to using children's pain relieving medicines, which you should use only under a doctor's instruction, you can place a warm (not hot) pad over the ear. Never put anything directly in the child's ear, including the safe, effective, and natural essential oil blends, unless specifically directed by a doctor.

Essential Oil Blends

Essential oils that assist in treating earaches are Basil, Chamomile (both Roman and German), Eucalyptus, Lavender, Peppermint, Rosemary, Tea Tree, and Thyme. Refer to the "Essential Oil Chart" for contraindications, warnings, or cautions about using essential oils.

We moved when my daughter was five years old. When her new doctor reviewed her previous medical records, she said, "You can't tell me that your child has never had an ear infection, can you?" When I explained that we have used aromatherapy products to provide a germ-free environment for her and that might explain it, the doctor's eyes glazed over and she smiled indulgently. If she wants to chalk it up to my child being one of the lucky few, so be it. I know better.

The Infant Earache Relief blend contains essential oils that are safe to use on infants as young as three-months old when used as directed.

Infant Earache Relief

6 drops Lavender

6 drops Tea Tree

4 drops Eucalyptus

> Add all of the essential oils to 2 tablespoons of olive oil. Apply a small amount of the blend to the cheekbones, behind the ear, down the side of the throat and across the half of the forehead on the side of the aching ear. Apply the blend 4 to 6 times a day until the earache subsides. You can expect relief within 3 - 5 days.

NOTE: Do NOT put the drops into the ear canal. You can put a few drops of the blend on a cotton ball and gently place that in the ear, but do not force the cotton ball into the ear canal.

Most of my clients who have benefited from these earache blends say, "I just wish I had known about aromatherapy when my older children were small. We had many ear infections and the worst part was not being able to ease their pain."

For children 2 years and up, the Toddler and Adult Earache Relief blend is safe and effective.

Toddler and Adult Earache Relief

4 drops Chamomile

3 drops Eucalyptus

4 drops Lavender

2 drops Peppermint

2 drops Rosemary

> Add all of the essential oils to 2 tablespoons of olive oil. Apply a small amount of the blend to the cheekbones, behind the ear, down the side of the throat and across the half of the forehead on the side of the aching ear. Apply the blend 4 to 6 times a day until the earache subsides. You can expect relief within 7 - 10 days.

Note: Do NOT put the drops into the ear canal. You can put a few drops of the blend on a cotton ball and gently place that in the ear, but do not force the cotton ball into the ear canal.

Flu

"From winter, plague and pestilence, good Lord, deliver us!"

Thomas Nash

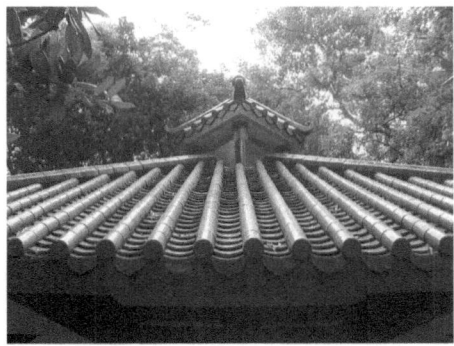

When the flu hits, you really do believe that only the Almighty can get you through the aches – even your hair hurts.

One of the most obvious characteristics of the flu is that it starts suddenly and hits hard. You'll probably feel weak and tired, and have a fever, dry cough, runny nose, chills, muscle aches, severe headache, eye pain, and a sore throat. You may wonder whether you have a cold or the flu. The symptoms are similar, but if you have severe symptoms, aching, and fever, you probably have the flu.

If you have the flu, there are things you can do to make yourself feel better. Stay home (the world can go on without you for a day or two) and rest, especially while you have a fever. Stop smoking and avoid secondhand smoke. Drink plenty of fluids like water, fruit juice, herbal tea, and clear soups. Avoid alcohol. Gargle with warm salt water a few times a day to relieve your sore throat. Throat sprays or lozenges may also help relieve the pain. Use salt water (saline) nose drops to help loosen mucus and moisten the tender skin in your nose.

You should contact your doctor if your flu lasts more than 3 days, or if you have a high fever, shortness of breath, wheezing, or a cough that just won't go away.

And don't forget the vitamin C. You can find it in orange juice and warm drinks, as well as in supplements. Also helpful are zinc lozenges – let them dissolve slowly in your mouth to let them reduce the duration of your symptoms. Echinacea is also helpful. Zinc and Echinacea should be taken when your immune system is under attack, but not routinely. As always, when taking supplements, read the label for any warnings or interactions.

Essential Oil Blends

The best essential oils for flu symptoms are Cinnamon, Eucalyptus, Lavender, Lemon, Peppermint, Rosemary, Tea Tree, and Thyme. Refer to the "Essential Oil Chart" for contraindications, warnings, or cautions about using essential oils.

When our next-door neighbor's child had the flu, my daughter and I made up this blend and took it to her along with some magazines. When my daughter saw her little friend lying in bed, shivering, with glazed eyes and pink cheeks, she was alarmed. I said, "Don't worry honey, your friend will get better. It's just that you have never had the flu and you are not familiar with what she is going through." Our neighbor was astounded that an 11-year old had never had the flu. I am convinced that using the blends in the "Infection" chapter on a regular basis has contributed to my daughter's flu-free life.

You will want to use the Flu Relief blend to ease your breathing, help your mucus clear, and keep the environment fresh and clean smelling.

Flu Relief

16 drops Eucalyptus

10 drops Lavender

6 drops Peppermint

6 drops Rosemary

> Mix all the oils together. Use in any or all of the following ways:
>
> Put 15 drops in a diffuser.
>
> Put 2 drops in a bath. Not only will the steam help clear out nasal passages, but also the calming properties of this blend will help your child rest.
>
> Add 15 drops to 2 teaspoons of carrier oil, and massage the child's lung area (chest and back).

Use the Flu Fighter blend for your sore or dry scratchy throat. Use this blend for several days after the major symptoms of flu are gone. The antiseptic properties of Lavender and Lemon help your body return to a healthy state and help you combat germs.

Years ago my doctor recommended a salt and baking soda gargle for a very sore throat. Adding the Lavender and Lemon essential oils helps it work better and faster. Plus, it is a bit more palatable.

Flu Fighter

2 drops Lavender

2 drops Lemon

> Add 1 teaspoon of salt, 1 teaspoon of baking soda, and the essential oils to a glass of warm water. Mix well. Gargle until it is all gone.

Headaches

"Pain and death are a part of life. To reject them is to reject life itself."

Havelock Ellis

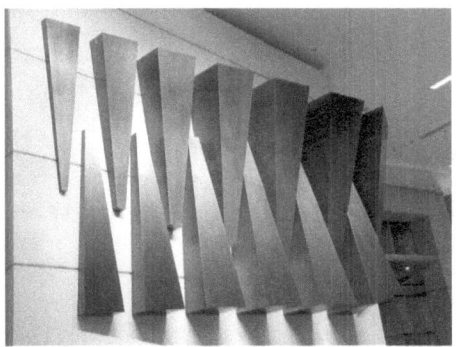

I could certainly reject the pain of headaches and not feel that I was rejecting life itself. The most difficult part of dealing with your headaches is figuring out the source of the headache. As you would with most physical ailments, eat properly, sleep sufficiently, exercise regularly, and make sure you have a stress-reducing hobby.

Over 90% of people experience some kind of headache. There are different kinds of head pain and they require different types of treatment. Proper diagnosis is essential to your overall health and is necessary to obtain the best possible treatment for your headaches. Here is a quick reference to some of the symptoms of common headaches:

Migraines:

- throbbing, intense pain, generally moderate to severe

- usually one-sided, pain is often near the eye of the affected side

- may last hours, days, or even weeks

- often accompanied by visual disturbances and/or extreme sensitivity to light, sound, and odors

Tension Headache:

- constant, dull pain, usually mild to moderate

- pain is often accompanied by muscle tightness in the shoulders and neck

- may last an hour, a week, or anywhere in between

Sinus/Allergy Headache:

- pain generally mild to moderate

- centered around sinuses, above and below eyes; pressure often makes teeth ache

- often seasonal

Cluster Headache:

- severely incapacitating sharp, stabbing pain; usually on one side of the head, centered around the eye; may also experience jaw, neck, and shoulder pain

- occur in clusters of 1 - 4 headaches a day for several days or weeks, lasting 10 minutes to two hours each, then stopping for months

- most frequent among men; in the fall and spring

Some Natural Suggestions

- Caffeine can cause headaches, but caffeine withdrawal can also cause headaches. Be moderate and consistent. You also might want to slowly substitute peppermint tea.

- Cayenne, used internally (add 1/8 to ½ teaspoon to half-cup of tomato juice or take cayenne capsules) is helpful for headaches caused by caffeine withdrawal.

- According to a University of Cincinnati study, fish oil (omega-3) can help prevent the onset and intensity of migraines in some cases.

Essential Oil Blends

Essential oils that assist in treating headaches are Basil, Chamomile (both Roman and German), Citronella, Clary Sage, Cumin, Eucalyptus, Grapefruit, Lavender, Lemon, Lemongrass, Marjoram, Peppermint, Rosemary, Rosewood, Sage, and Thyme. Refer to the "Essential Oil Chart" for contraindications, warnings, or cautions about using essential oils.

The Headache Relief blend contains essential oils that have anti-inflammatory and sedative properties. This blend helps soothe, calm, and relieve your pain.

I have heard that water and oxygen are the two greatest relievers of headaches. When headache strikes, during the 20 minutes that you are using the compress blends below, drink plenty of water, breathe deeply, and relax your muscles.

Headache Relief

4 drops Chamomile

4 drops Lavender

2 drops Peppermint

2 drops Rosemary

> Mix all the oils together in a dark glass container. Put 3 drops of the essential oil blend on a cool damp towel. Lie down and place the cool compress on your forehead. Rest for about 20 minutes.

> Add the remaining essential oils to 2 tablespoons of carrier oil (any oil listed in the "Carrier Oils" chapter). Shake well and rub the base of your neck 4 to 6 times until the headache goes away.

The Headache Soother blend seems to work better on stress-related headaches.

Headache Soother

2 drops Clary Sage

4 drops Grapefruit

4 drops Lemon

4 drops Marjoram

> Mix all the oils together in a dark glass container. Put 3 drops of the essential oil blend on a cool damp towel. Lie down and place the cool compress on your forehead. Rest for about 20 minutes.

> Add the remaining essential oils to 2 tablespoons of base carrier oil (any oil listed in the "Carrier Oils" chapter). Shake well and rub the base of your neck 4 to 6 times until the headache goes away.

Immune System

"If you think you are beaten, you are.
If you think that you dare not, you don't.
If you'd like to win, but you think you can't.
It's almost certain you won't."

Anonymous

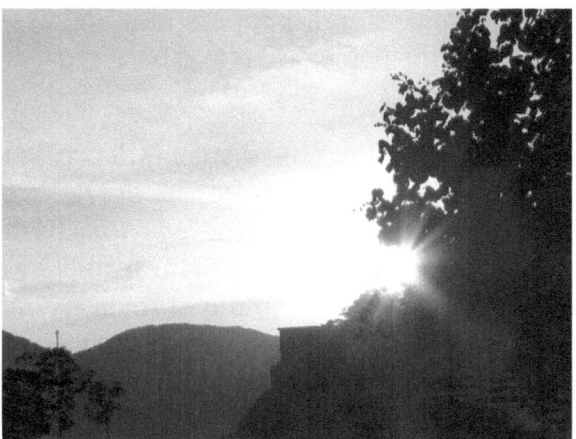

Negative mental attitude, as the quotation suggests, results in negative outcomes. Not a surprise. Using the same logic, a positive mental attitude goes a long way to achieving positive results. Combine a positive mental attitude with the power of a strong immune system and you can take on just about anything.

The immune system is a fascinating and complex system composed of many interdependent cell types that collectively protect the body from bacterial, parasitic, fungal, and viral infections and from the growth of tumor cells. It is worth your time to investigate as much about the immune system as you can, as it is the core of your health. While extensive details about the immune system are beyond the scope of this book, here are some highlights. All the cells of the immune system initially come from the bone marrow. The function of the thymus is to produce mature T cells that are then released into the bloodstream. In the spleen, while old blood cells are destroyed, B cells become activated and produce large amounts of antibodies. Lymph nodes, found throughout the body, drain fluid from most of your tissues.

There will be times that you feel your immune system is depressed and needs an extra boost to help bring you to a better state of health. At those times, you want an immune stimulant. However, long term use of an immune stimulant robs your body of its natural ability to be at a state of health, so you want to use an immune stimulant only for a limited time (3 – 7 days). The rest of the time you can use an immune system tonic to support your immune system.

This is how I explain the difference between a stimulant and a tonic to my clients. Suppose I was tutoring you in math, in the beginning I am doing all of the work because the material is completely new to you and you are deficient. That's the role of the stimulant. However, once you start catching on, I want you to do as much of the math work on your own as you can, and just provide a constant low-level amount of support. That's the role of the tonic. In the end you are going to successfully pass that math test on your own, and that's the goal of overall good health.

Essential Oil Blends

The best essential oils for your immune system are grouped into immune system tonics and immune system stimulants. Immune system tonic oils are: Basil, Cedarwood, Chamomile, Frankincense, Myrrh, Patchouli, Rosewood, Sandalwood, Spruce, Yarrow, and Ylang Ylang. Immune system stimulant oils are: Black Pepper, Cinnamon, Clove, Eucalyptus, Lemon, Lemongrass, Nutmeg,

Pine, Tea Tree, and Vetiver. Refer to the "Essential Oil Chart" for contraindications, warnings, or cautions about using essential oils.

It's cold and flu season; you are going on a field trip with a roomful of children; you are under a great deal of stress; you are traveling a lot. If any of these scenarios apply to you, now is a good time for an Immune System Stimulant.

Immune System Stimulant – Teens and Adults

8 drops Cinnamon

8 drops Clove

10 drops Tea Tree

> Add all essential oils to 2 tablespoons of carrier oil (any oil listed in the "Carrier Oils" chapter). Shake well and dab on your pulse points and on the base of your neck 4 to 6 times daily during the period of time in which you want to boost your immune system.

While I wholeheartedly believe that a good diet, plenty of rest, an appropriate amount of exercise, and sufficient relaxation time are all necessary to keep a child happy and healthy, there are times when their bodies need an extra boost to fight off germs. This is the perfect time for the Immune System Stimulant for Children.

Immune System Stimulant – Children

10 drops Eucalyptus

8 drops Lemon

8 drops Tea Tree

> Add all essential oils to 2 tablespoons of carrier oil (any oil listed in the "Carrier Oils" chapter). Shake well and dab onto pulse points and the base of the neck 4 to 6 times daily during the period of time in which you want to boost your immune system.

You really want your immune system to work at its maximum level at all times. However, our bodies are battered daily by pollutants, stress, improper diet, and so much more, that it makes sense to give your immune system some gentle support on a daily basis. The Immune System Tonic fulfills that need and happens to have some essential oils that are good for your skin and your emotional state as well.

Immune System Tonic

5 drops Chamomile

5 drops Patchouli

5 drops Rosewood

5 drops Spruce

> Add all essential oils to 2 tablespoons of carrier oil (any oil listed in the "Carrier Oils" chapter). Shake well and dab on your pulse points and on the base of your neck 4 to 6 times daily during the period of time in which you want to support your immune system.

Indigestion

"It's not what you're eating, it's what's eating you."

Janet Greeson

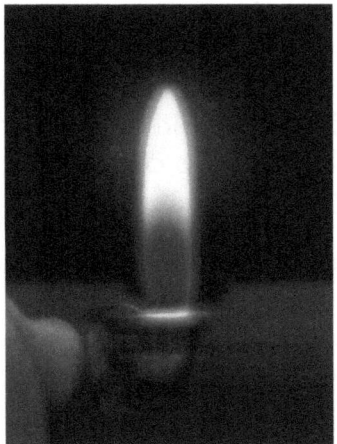

That quotation really captures how you feel when you have indigestion. Whether it is from overeating during the holidays, over indulging on junk food, or excessive use of alcohol, we can all probably say, "been there, done that, didn't like it."

Indigestion is discomfort or a burning sensation in the upper abdomen (also called heartburn), often accompanied by nausea, abdominal bloating, belching, and sometimes vomiting.

For many people, indigestion results from eating too much, eating too quickly, eating high-fat foods, or eating during stressful situations. Smoking, drinking too much alcohol, using medications that irritate the stomach lining, being tired, and having ongoing stress can also cause indigestion or make it worse.

Avoiding the foods and situations that seem to cause indigestion can be the most successful way to avoid it. Also, take your time while you eat, chew food carefully and thoroughly, and avoid conflicts at meals. Peppermint tea or ginger tea can be helpful in dealing with the symptoms of indigestion.

Because indigestion can mimic a more serious disease, see a doctor if you have:

- Vomiting, weight loss, or appetite loss

- Black tarry stools or blood in vomit

- Severe pain in the upper right abdomen (if severe pain is in the lower right abdomen, check with your physician for possible appendicitis).

- Discomfort unrelated to eating

- Shortness of breath, sweating, or pain radiating to the jaw, neck, or arm

Essential Oil Blends

The best essential oils for indigestion and heartburn are Clove, Eucalyptus, Fennel, Ginger, Lavender, and Peppermint. Refer to the "Essential Oil Chart" for contraindications, warnings, or cautions about using essential oils.

For many of my clients who suffer from indigestion, the most effective long-term treatment is to avoid those stressors that cause the indigestion. I frequently suggest to people that they keep a diary of their lifestyle and habits for about one week. When you take a look at this diary you can pinpoint the elements in your life that you must change and start creating a plan for better health.

When the pain and burning of indigestion is just too much to bear, use the Intense Indigestion Relief blend. The pain relieving properties of the essential oils will ease inflammation, provide analgesic support, and quiet your discomfort.

Intense Indigestion Relief

10 drops Chamomile

8 drops Juniper

8 drops Lavender

8 drops Peppermint

> Add the essential oils to 4 ounces of base lotion or 4 tablespoons of carrier oil (any oil listed in the "Carrier Oils" chapter). **Gently** apply a small amount of the blend to the abdomen and to the lower back around the kidney area in soft, circular motions. Apply the blend 4 to 6 times a day until the indigestion subsides. You can expect relief within 1 - 3 days.

Ginger and Fennel are both used for digestive problems. The Irritating Indigestion Soother blend is great when constipation or irritable bowels are also symptoms of your indigestion.

Irritating Indigestion Soother

8 drops Bergamot

8 drops Fennel

8 drops Ginger

10 drops Peppermint

> Add the essential oils to 4 ounces of base lotion or 4 tablespoons of carrier oil (any oil listed in the "Carrier Oils" chapter). **Gently** apply a small amount of the blend to the abdomen and to the lower back around the kidney area in soft, circular motions. Apply the blend 4 to 6 times a day until the indigestion subsides. You can expect relief within 1 - 3 days.

"Push back from the table," is probably my most common statement to people who suffer from indigestion. I would rather ask for a doggy bag for those extra rich foods that you don't want to eat all at the same time, than suffer from indigestion.

After you treat the significant symptoms of indigestion, use the Indigestion Comforter for several days to assist your system in returning to a normal – and more comfortable – state.

Indigestion Comforter

8 drops Ginger

8 drops Lemon

10 drops Peppermint

> Add the essential oils to 4 ounces of base lotion or 4 tablespoons of carrier oil (any oil listed in the "Carrier Oils" chapter). **Gently** apply a small amount of the blend to the abdomen and to the lower back around the kidney area in soft, circular motions. Apply the blend 4 to 6 times a day until the indigestion subsides. You can expect relief within 1 - 3 days.

Sinus Problems

"No warmth, no cheerfulness, no helpful ease."

Thomas Hood

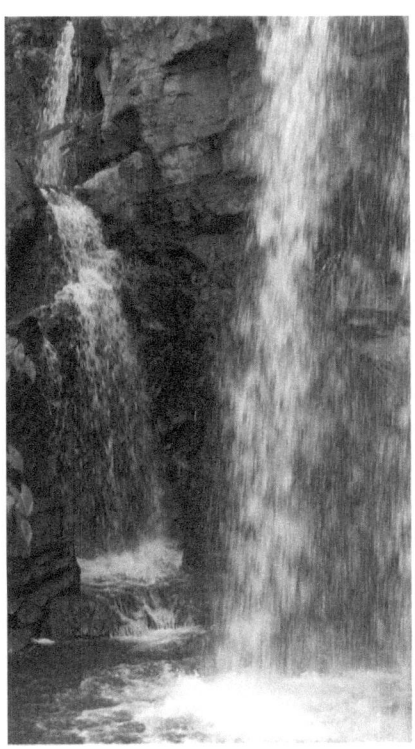

Got a big head filled with cement? Does it feel like some phantom is pressing down on your nose until you can't even breathe? You could be feeling sinus pressure. Use the essential oil blends to get cheerfulness and helpful ease.

All sorts of advertisements talk about the pain or pressure in some areas of the face (forehead, cheeks, or between the eyes), stuffy nose, fever, and nasal mucus. And, millions of dollars are spent each year in trying to treat sinus problems. There are many causes of sinus discomfort including changes in temperature or air pressure, smoking, bacterial or viral infection, overuse of nasal sprays, swimming, diving, or having growths called polyps blocking your sinus passages.

Most people know about the sinus chambers behind the cheeks, eyebrows, and jaw, but there are also areas at the base of the skull and behind the ears that when inflamed can cause sinus discomfort. In fact, if you suffer from sinus headaches, check the sinus pockets at the base of your skull — they will be puffy and enlarged. If you get postnasal drip, check the sinus pockets behind your ears.

There are some things that you can do to help yourself feel better. Get lots of rest. Drink plenty of fluids. Apply moist heat by holding a warm, wet towel against your face or breathing in steam through a cloth or towel. Rinse your sinus passages with a saline solution. One of the things you'll want to do is get that mucus moving. Hot spicy food, such as salsa, horseradish, and wasabi, to name a few, can be very helpful to make your nose run. Don't forget the tried and true bowl of peppery chicken soup.

If your problem persists for more than 3 days, you should consult your doctor who can explore over-the-counter products, antibiotics, or other treatment options.

Essential Oil Blends

The best essential oils for upper respiratory issues are Clove, Cypress, Eucalyptus, Lavender, Peppermint, Pine, Rosemary, and Tea Tree. Refer to the "Essential Oil Chart" for contraindications, warnings, or cautions about using essential oils.

The following aromatherapy blends can be used as either inhalants or massage blends. Let your personal preference guide you. The Man's Man Sinus Treatment blend is extremely effective and preferred by my man — maybe it's the rugged outdoor smell of the pine.

The Man's Man Sinus Treatment

80 drops Eucalyptus

100 drops Pine

80 drops Tea Tree

> Mix all the oils together in a dark glass container. There is so much you can do with these oils.

Lotion

> Add 25 drops of the essential oils to 4 ounces of base lotion or 4 tablespoons of carrier oil (any oil listed in the "Carrier Oils" chapter). Apply a small amount of the blend:

> At least 5-6 times per day for the first three days, then you can reduce it to at least twice a day.

> - If you suffer sinus headaches, apply the blend to the nape of your neck.
>
> - If you suffer from post nasal drip, apply the blend behind your ears.
>
> - If you have nasal congestion, apply the blend on your cheeks, below your nose, on your forehead, and put a little at the base of your nose so you can breathe in the relief.
>
> - For bronchial congestion, apply the blend to the chest and back (lung area).

> You only need a tiny amount. If you massage the cream onto the affected area three times and you still see the lotion, you have used too much. The beauty of essential oils is that they are very concentrated, so you only need a little bit. The lotion is there only to apply the oils to your skin so that the oils can be absorbed into the bloodstream. Start with a tiny amount, you can always put on a little more.

As is also true for any prescribed medication for sinus relief, this essential oil protocol does NOT work after just one application. You must use the blend regularly for at least one week to start noticing an improvement. If the first time you use the blend, your nose starts running quite a bit, let it – this is a good thing.

Vaporizer Blend (see information about vaporizers in the "Introduction" chapter)

Add 15 to 30 drops of the blend to the water in your vaporizer. Day 1 – fill vaporizer and put in 15 drops of oils. Day 2 – just refill the water to the top (that is if the water reduces about 1/3 of the way). Day 3 – just refill the water to the top (that is if the water reduces about 1/3 of the way). Day 4 – empty vaporizer, clean it out, and start at Day 1 again.

Note: Some vaporizers use up all of the water overnight. If that happens with yours then you need to add clean water and new drops each day. In that case, you can use just 10 drops each night. You will still want to wash out the vaporizer after 4 days.

Inhaler

You can use this blend as an inhaler. Simply inhale the aroma of the oils from the bottle (take 3 long "belly breaths" each time you inhale). Do NOT apply the oils directly to the skin.

Room Spray

Put 28 drops of the blend in one cup of water. Put that into a spray bottle and spray your room, office, car, etc. regularly.

House Cleaner

Put 22 drops of the blend in a quart of water. Shake well, and spray. This can clean EVERYTHING in your house. You can also use 22 drops of the blend in the washing machine for each load of clothes and in the dishwasher to wash your dishes.

One of the outstanding features of essential oils is that they have many chemical properties. In the Ladies' Preferred Sinus Treatment, we use Geranium for its natural expectorant properties. Geranium is also helpful in balancing hormones. Rosemary is another essential oil that resonates with women. In this blend it is used for its antibacterial properties.

Ladies Preferred Sinus Treatment

32 drops Eucalyptus

80 drops Geranium

48 drops Peppermint

80 drops Rosemary

> Mix all the oils together in a dark glass container. There is so much you can do with these oils.

Lotion

> Add 25 drops of the essential oils to 4 ounces of base lotion or 4 tablespoons of carrier oil (any oil listed in the "Carrier Oils" chapter). Apply a small amount of the blend:
>
> At least 5-6 times per day for the first three days, then you can reduce it to at least twice a day.
>
> - If you suffer sinus headaches, apply the blend to the nape of your neck.
>
> - If you suffer from post nasal drip, apply the blend behind your ears.
>
> - If you have nasal congestion, apply the blend on your cheeks, below your nose, on your forehead, and put a little at the base of your nose so you can breathe in the relief.
>
> - For bronchial congestion, apply the blend to the chest and back (lung area).
>
> You only need a tiny amount. If you massage the cream onto the affected area three times and you still see the lotion, you have used too much. The beauty of essential oils is that they are very concentrated, so you only need a little bit. The lotion is there only to apply the oils to your skin so that the oils can be absorbed into the bloodstream. Start with a tiny amount, you can always put on a little more.

As is also true for any prescribed medication for sinus relief, this essential oil protocol does NOT work after just one application. You must use the blend regularly for at least one week to start noticing an improvement. If the first time you use the blend, your nose starts running quite a bit, let it – this is a good thing.

Vaporizer Blend (see information about vaporizers in the "Introduction" chapter)

Add 15 to 30 drops of the blend to the water in your vaporizer. Day 1 – fill vaporizer and put in 15 drops of oils. Day 2 – just refill the water to the top (that is if the water reduces about 1/3 of the way). Day 3 – just refill the water to the top (that is if the water reduces about 1/3 of the way). Day 4 – empty vaporizer, clean it out, and start at Day 1 again.

Note: Some vaporizers use up all of the water overnight. If that happens with yours then you need to add clean water and new drops each day. In that case, you can use just 10 drops each night. You will still want to wash out the vaporizer after 4 days.

Inhaler

You can use this blend as an inhaler. Simply inhale the aroma of the oils from the bottle (take 3 long "belly breaths" each time you inhale). Do NOT apply the oils directly to the skin.

Room Spray

Put 28 drops of the blend in one cup of water. Put that into a spray bottle and spray your room, office, car, etc. regularly.

House Cleaner

Put 22 drops of the blend in a quart of water. Shake well, and spray. This can clean EVERYTHING in your house. You can also use 22 drops of the blend in the washing machine for each load of clothes and in the dishwasher to wash your dishes.

The Kid's Sinus Treatment is effective for children age 3 and older.

My daughter suffers from seasonal allergies, so I always have the Kid's Sinus Treatment blend in my home. The first thing I recommend to all of my sinus clients is to get rid of synthetic house cleaners or room sprays. When your respiratory and bronchial area is already under stress, you want to avoid anything that is going to aggravate it further. Many of my clients have found that using the natural House Cleaner blend described in the instructions under the first blend is the ONLY thing they needed to do to help relieve their child's stuffiness.

Kid's Sinus Treatment

60 drops Eucalyptus

80 drops Lavender

60 drops Pine

60 drops Tea Tree

Lotion

> Add 25 drops of the essential oils to 4 ounces of base lotion or 4 tablespoons of base carrier oil (any oil listed in the "Carrier Oils" chapter). Apply a small amount of the blend to the chest and back (lung area) at least 5-6 times per day for the first three days, then you can reduce it to at least twice a day.

Vaporizer Blend (see information about vaporizers in the "Introduction" chapter)

> Add 15 to 30 drops of the blend to the water in your vaporizer. Day 1 – fill vaporizer and put in 15 drops of oils. Day 2 – just refill the water to the top (that is if the water reduces about 1/3 of the way). Day 3 – just refill the water to the top (that is if the water reduces about 1/3 of the way). Day 4 – empty vaporizer, clean it out, and start at Day 1 again.

Note: Some vaporizers use up all of the water up overnight. If that happens with yours then you need to add clean water and new drops each day. In that is the case, you can just use 10 drops each night. You will still want to wash out the vaporizer after 4 days.

First Aid

What do I need in a first aid kit?

The American Red Cross suggests the following items for your first aid kit: (20) adhesive bandages, various sizes, (1) 5" x 9" sterile dressing, (1) conforming roller gauze bandage, (2) triangular bandages, (2) 3 x 3 sterile gauze pads, (2) 4 x 4 sterile gauze pads, (1) roll 3" cohesive bandage, (2) germicidal hand wipes or waterless alcohol-based hand sanitizer, (6) antiseptic wipes, (2) pair large medical grade non-latex gloves, adhesive tape, 2" width, antibacterial ointment, cold pack, scissors (small, personal), tweezers, and CPR breathing barrier, such as a face shield.

Please note that you can make a germicidal hand wipe, hand sanitizer, antiseptic wipes, and antibacterial ointment using essential oils. See the recipes in the "Infection" chapter.

The remainder of this section deals with:

- Bruises
- Burns
- Cuts and Scrapes
- Infection
- Inflammation
- Insect Bites and Repellent
- Poison Ivy and Itching
- Sunburn

Bruises

"Never a lip is curved with pain that can't be kissed into smiles again."

Bret Harte

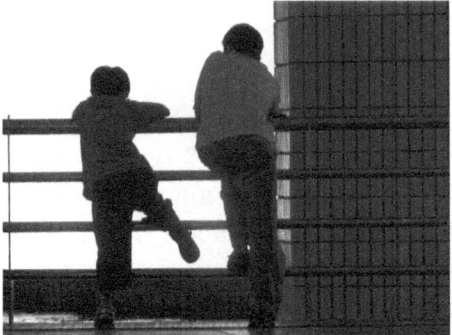

It seems that a parent's kiss is the cure for just about every childhood ailment, especially bruises. Bruises are typically not a serious condition — they go away relatively quickly on their own. Perhaps a kiss is just what this kind of boo-boo requires.

A bruise, also called a contusion, occurs when the soft tissues under your skin are injured: small veins and capillaries break and leak out red blood cells. It is these blood cells that cause that bluish, purplish, reddish, or blackish marks. That's where black-and-blue marks get their name — from the appearance they give to skin. As the body tries to heal itself from a bruise, you may have increased blood supply which causes a form of congestion which may cause swelling, tenderness, pain, heat, and redness.

If the skin isn't broken, a bandage isn't necessary. You can enhance healing by: elevating the injured area, applying ice or a cold pack for 30 to 60 minutes at a time for a day or two after the injury, and increasing your intake of vitamin C. Most bruises will disappear after 2 weeks — some will go away even sooner.

If a bruise does not go away after 2 weeks, you may want to let your doctor know. You should also contact your doctor if: you have unusually large or painful bruises, especially if there seems to be no reason for the bruise; you bruise easily and you're experiencing abnormal bleeding elsewhere, such as from your nose or gums; you notice blood in your eyes or your urine; or if you have no history of bruising but suddenly experience bruises.

Essential Oil Blends

Essential oils that can help with bruises are Black Pepper, Chamomile, Clove, Cypress, Geranium, Lavender, Marjoram, Peppermint, Rosemary, and Thyme. Refer to the "Essential Oil Chart" for contraindications, warnings, or cautions about using essential oils.

To treat bruises, muscle aches, or sprains anywhere on your body, apply the essential oil blends in a straight upward motion; see the "Aches & Pains" section for details.

When you first get a bruise, your first steps should be to reduce the swelling and relieve the pain. The Bruise Reducer is a great blend to achieve both of those results.

Bruise Reducer

8 drops Chamomile

6 drops Cypress

6 drops Geranium

2 drops Peppermint

> Mix all the oils together in a dark glass container. For the first 48 hours, apply a cold compress to the affected area as often as possible, up to 3 times per hour. Place 3 drops of the blend onto the cold wet cloth before each application. Keep the compress on the affected area until the cloth reaches room temperature.
>
> After 48 hours, add the remainder of the essential oil blend to 2 ounces of base lotion or 2 tablespoons carrier oil (any oil listed in the "Carrier Oils" chapter). Apply a small amount of the blend to the area of injury and the areas immediately above and below the site of injury. Apply the blend 4 to 6 times a day for the first 3 – 5 days until the pain subsides.

Once the swelling has been reduced and the pain is diminished, you want to draw out any congestion and increase the circulation of blood to continue healing the area. Clove and Cypress in the Bruise Soother blend help draw out congestion while the other ingredients promote healing.

Bruise Soother

4 drops Black Pepper

4 drops Clove

6 drops Cypress

6 drops Marjoram

4 drops Peppermint

4 drops Rosemary

> Add all the oils to 2 ounces of base lotion or 2 tablespoons carrier oil (any oil listed in the "Carrier Oils" chapter). Apply a small amount of the blend to the area of injury and the areas immediately above and below the site of injury. Apply the blend 4 to 6 times a day for the first 3 – 5 days until the pain subsides.

Use the Bruise Assistance blend to promote health on the inside and outside of the bruised area.

When my daughter was younger and I would kiss away her "owies," she would hold my face in her hands, examine my lips, and very seriously ask, "Do you have Vavender [Lavender] and Uranium [Geranium] in there?"

Bruise Assistance

10 drops Geranium

10 drops Lavender

8 drops Rosemary

5 drops Thyme

> Add all the oils to 2 ounces of base lotion or 2 tablespoons carrier oil (any oil listed in the "Carrier Oils" chapter). Apply a small amount of the blend to the area of injury and the areas immediately above and below the site of injury. Apply the blend 4 to 6 times a day for the first 3 – 5 days until the pain subsides.

Burns

"Fire answers fire."

Shakespeare

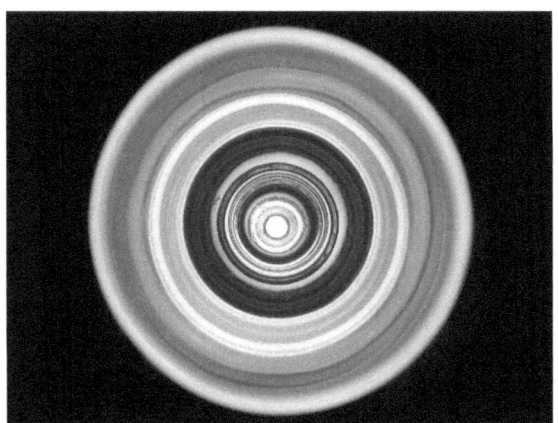

You got just a bit too close to the flame and you will feel that fire for days. Whether it was from a cooking accident, loading the wood stove carelessly, steam from the iron, or hot wax from a spilled candle, you have a burn. Or your child has a burn. Essential oils are extremely effective for offering not only temporary relief from the pain of the burn, but also lasting relief to heal the skin.

Burns are a common occurrence in our lives – from sunburn to a burn from scalding water. There are actually three degrees of burns. Identifying burns properly is the first step towards treating them appropriately. First-degree burns, most sunburns and scalds, are red and painful. Second degree burns, severe sunburns or burns caused by brief contact with flames, blister, ooze, and are very painful.

Many doctors agree that you can treat most first and second degree burns yourself. To do so, run cold tap water directly onto the burn for at least 20 minutes. Never use ice. Ice damages the delicate, and now injured, tissue. You can put a cool compress on the burn. Make sure you change it frequently to keep the cool temperature on the affected area.

Third degree burns are an entirely different story. Third degree burns require medical attention immediately. Third degree burns are charred, white, or creamy colored. They can be caused by chemicals, electricity, fire, or prolonged contact with hot surfaces. Usually they are not painful because nerve endings have been destroyed.

You also want to contact a doctor if a burn shows a sign of infection (blister filled with greenish/brownish fluid), if the burn is on a sensitive part of your body, or if the burn doesn't heal within 10 days.

As you treat the burn and as it heals, keep it clean, dry, and protected from bumping. Don't bandage the burn — you want air to help in the healing process. If you have a burn that seems to require a bandage, you should probably see your doctor about that burn. This would also be a good time to up your intake of vitamin C, which is helpful against both the inflammation of the burn and any infection.

Essential Oil Blends

The best essential oils for healing and rejuvenating your skin are Carrot, Chamomile, Clary Sage, Frankincense, Geranium, Lavender, Peppermint, and Rosemary. Refer to the "Essential Oil Chart" for contraindications, warnings, or cautions about using essential oils.

The quickest, best emergency treatment for a burn is plain Lavender essential oil. Apply drops of Lavender directly to the burn.

An interesting bit of history, it all started with a burn. René-Maurice Gattefossé is considered the father of the term "aromatherapy." He was a French perfumist who one day while practicing his trade, burned his arm over a flame. Without thinking, he stuck his arm in a vat of Lavender essential oil, which he was using to make perfume. When his arm healed quickly, he decided that Lavender had both aroma and therapy. Now you know.

As the burn heals, the skin in and around it may feel itchy. This is often a sign of healing. Use one of the blends below to heal the burn and soothe the skin. The Burn Soother blend is great for anyone of any age. If you are treating a very young child (under 2 years) or a pregnant woman, use the Chamomile and Lavender; Peppermint is just a bit too harsh.

Burn Soother

6 drops Chamomile

6 drops Lavender OR 6 drops of Peppermint

> Use a palmful (approximately one tablespoon) of hand cream, carrier oil, or (since this is an emergency) water or milk. Add the essential oils, mix together, and apply to the burn often.

> You can also mix up a small batch of this (in a container, not in your hand) and use it on the burn whenever it feels dry or itchy. You can expect relief within 3 – 5 days.

The Burn Relief blend is a "must have" in your first aid kit. Chamomile is an anti-inflammatory; Geranium rejuvenates damaged skin cells; Peppermint aids in keeping the site antiseptically clean and helps with the itch and pain; while the Lavender is a terrific soother.

Burn Relief

16 drops Chamomile

8 drops Geranium

20 drops Lavender

4 drops Peppermint

Mix all the oils together in a dark glass container.

For use in the first 48 hours, make a cooling spray by putting 24 drops of the combined blend in 8 ounces of cold water in a spray bottle. Keep this refrigerated. Spray on the affected area as often as possible, up to 3 times per hour.

After 48 hours, add the remainder of the essential oils to 2 tablespoons of one of the carrier oils. Use a cotton ball to absorb a small amount of this blend and then squeeze the cotton ball to drop the blend onto the burn and the areas immediately above and below the site of injury. You could also use a dropper. Apply this blend 4 to 6 times a day for the first 3 – 5 days until the burn subsides.

Cuts and Scrapes

"This was the most unkindest cut of all."

William Shakespeare

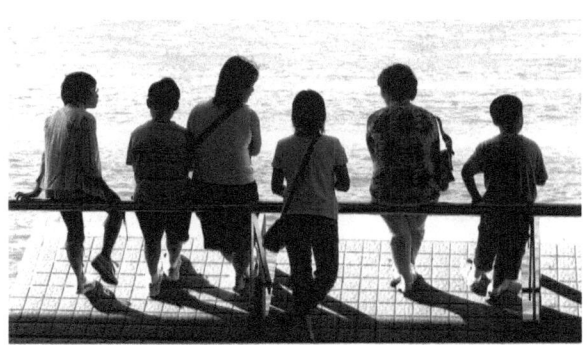

I wanted to name this chapter, Boo-boos, because everyone knows what they are. It didn't sound serious enough, or grown up enough, or something. I hate acting grown up, but I want to present information about essential oils in a pragmatic and realistic way. Just because my daughter and I had a water gun fight and ate ice cream before I started working for the day, it shouldn't take away from the serious value that essential oils offer.

A wound is a break in the skin. It can also be called a cut, scrape, laceration, gash, or tear. Some are minor and can be easily treated at home, while others may need stitches to heal. The greatest concern you have with a cut or scrape is keeping the germs out to prevent infection.

For minor cuts and scrapes, wash the affected area with cool water and soap, and then cover with a light protective adhesive bandage. Keep the injured area and dressing dry and check daily for signs of infection, such as fever, red streaks around the cut, or yellowish/greenish liquid oozing from the cut. While the use of an over-the-counter antibiotic or antiseptic is optional, you should avoid using alcohol.

If you child complains of numbness or that the cut hurts more, or you can feel that the affected area is warm or swollen, consult your doctor.

Essential Oil Blends

The best essential oils for healing skin and fighting infection are Chamomile, Geranium, Lavender, Rosemary, and Tea Tree. Refer to the "Essential Oil Chart" for contraindications, warnings, or cautions about using essential oils.

The recipes below give you directions for creating a spray (very nice since you don't have to touch the wound to apply the blend) and a lotion (either oil base or lotion base). The Cuts and Scrapes Relief blend is ideal for several reasons. The Tea Tree has antiseptic, anti-fungal, antibacterial properties to clean and keep germs away. The Chamomile is an anti-inflammatory to ease pain and lessen swelling. The Geranium contains properties that heal damaged cells and the Lavender is soothing.

As a soccer coach for my daughter's team, I always carry the Cuts and Scrapes Relief blend in my bag. One of my players got a pretty nasty cut complete with ground-in dirt and grass. Her parents skeptically looked on while I applied the blend and were amazed that it didn't sting and, before practice was over, you could see a noticeable improvement.

Cuts and Scrapes Relief

15 drops Chamomile

10 drops Geranium

15 drops Lavender

12 drops Tea Tree

> Mix all the oils together in a dark glass container.
>
> Add 22 drops of the blended oils to 8 ounces of water in a spray bottle. When a cut or scrape occurs, cleanse the wound with this blend.
>
> Add 30 drops of the essential oils to 4 ounces of base lotion or 4 tablespoons of base oil (any oil listed in the "Carrier Oils" chapter). Apply a small amount of the blend to the affected area 4 to 6 times a day until the wound heals.

The following blend is best used for soaking the wounded area, but you could also use it in a water-based spray. *People have frequently asked me, "If you could have only one or two essential oils, which ones would they be?" I always respond, "Lavender and Tea Tree. Between those two oils, you can treat many ailments for young and old alike."*

Cuts and Scrapes Soother

14 drops Lavender

6 drops Tea Tree

> Add 4 drops of Tea Tree and 10 drops of Lavender to 2 cups warm water to bathe the wound.
>
> Apply 2 drops of Tea Tree and 4 drops of Lavender directly to the boo-boo.

Infection

"The art of medicine consists of amusing the patient while nature cures the disease."

Voltaire

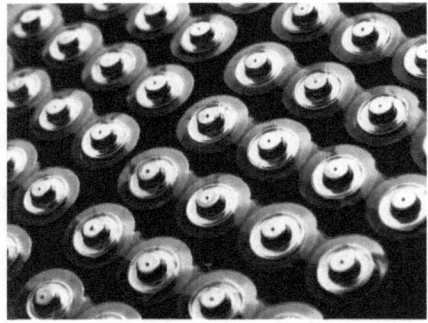

What a wonderful sentiment, but when you have a child home ill due to an infection, keeping the patient amused can be a difficult task. I remember when I was a child my mother would get an old 3-ring binder, lined paper, pencils, and crayons. She would then cut out puzzles from the newspaper, or make up pages of age-appropriate activities to keep me from getting bored when I was home sick.

Most research about infection links it to a particular part of the body, such as vaginal infections, bladder infections, infectious hepatitis, and so on. You also have viral infections and bacterial infections. The precautions that you are frequently given, such as washing your hands regularly and avoiding germ-filled environments, are almost impossible outside of a bubble. The best thing you can do with an infection is to avoid it. You want to diffuse and apply antibacterial and antiseptic essential oils on a regular basis to protect yourself and your family against infection.

At a recent seminar I asked the room full of mothers how often their children had stayed home from school in the past three months due to illness. The numbers were staggering. What was probably more unbelievable to this audience was that my then 11-year-old daughter had only missed a handful of school days due to illness during her entire school career. How is that possible? Since she was first exposed to daycare, I sprayed her body with the Antiseptic Spray recipe here. Can I absolutely prove that was the sole reason for her good health? Maybe not, but ask any mother, and she'll say, "I'll try it."

Essential Oil Blends

The best essential oils for infections are Cinnamon, Eucalyptus, Geranium, Lavender, Lemon, Pine, Tea Tree, and Thyme. Refer to the "Essential Oil Chart" for contraindications, warnings, or cautions about using essential oils.

Germ carriers are everywhere! For decades we have been advised to wash our hands regularly and disinfect every surface we encounter to avoid germs. Millions of dollars have been spent on germ fighters for every inch of our homes, cars, offices, and bodies. But for just pennies a day you can make your own (second to none) germ-fighting blend. If you are going to spray the Antiseptic Spray blend on children under the age of five, spray the bottom of their feet. This way they won't inadvertently touch the blend, then rub their eyes.

The Antiseptic Spray is safe enough to spray all over your body so you can put up a barrier between you and the germs of the world.

Antiseptic Spray

6 drops Eucalyptus

8 drops Lavender

7 drops Lemon

4 drops Rosemary

4 drops Tea Tree

> Add all drops of the blend to 1 quart of water. Use this as a spray to clean floors and other surfaces; disinfect germ-prone areas such as toys, telephones, and light switches; and cleanse every nook and cranny, calming and cleaning as you go.

The Infection Relief blend is strong and effective. Follow the instructions to make the blend as a spray and spritz the area to cleanse the infection. Then, follow the instructions to mix with a carrier oil for ongoing protection.

Infection Relief

8 drops Cinnamon

12 drops Eucalyptus

15 drops Lemon

12 drops Tea Tree

12 drops Thyme

> Mix all the oils together in a dark glass container.
>
> Put 29 drops of the blended oils in 8 ounces of water in a spray bottle. When an infection occurs, cleanse the infected area with this blend.
>
> Add 30 drops of the essential oils to 4 ounces of base lotion or 4 tablespoons of carrier oil (any oil listed in the "Carrier Oils" chapter). Apply a small amount of the blend to the affected area 4 to 6 times a day until the infection heals. You can expect relief within 3 - 5 days.

Note: Use extra caution with Cinnamon essential oil, it should never be allowed to touch your skin straight from the bottle.

Inflammation

"There are only two ways to live your life. One is as though nothing is a miracle. The other is as though everything is a miracle."

Albert Einstein

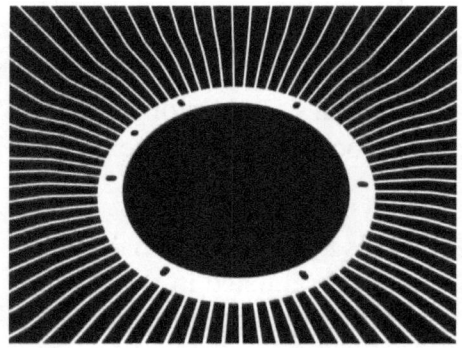

I hope that by this point in the book you realize that essential oils can offer miraculous benefits to your overall health and well-being. Whether you are treating an common ailment, such as inflammation, or something more elusive, such as emotional concerns, essential oils offer support, assistance, and, in some cases, miracles.

Inflammation is localized redness, warmth, swelling, and pain resulting from infection, irritation, or injury. Inflammation is your body's response to damage. It brings your natural defenses to the site of injury and removes bacteria and toxins from the damaged area. If your inflammation is accompanied by pus or blood, you should see your physician as soon as possible.

Inflammation can be acute or chronic. Acute inflammation is short lasting — lasting only a few days. When it is longer lasting it is referred to as chronic inflammation. Acute inflammation may be due to physical damage, chemical substances, bacteria, poor diet, or hormonal imbalance. Examples of acute inflammation are sore throat, skin reactions to a scratch or insect bite, and any kind of burn. If you have chronic inflammation, see your physician who can request diagnostic tests to help identify the cause of your chronic inflammation.

Vitamin C has natural anti-inflammatory properties. You may also find over-the-counter anti-inflammatories such as aspirin and ibuprophen helpful at this time. Ask your doctor about this.

Other chapters that deal with various kinds of inflammation are "Burns," "Dermatitis," "Diaper Rash," "Insect Bites and Repellent," "Poison Ivy and Itching," "Rash," "Shaving and Razor Burn", and "Sunburn".

Essential Oil Blends

Essential oils that can help ease inflammation are Cedarwood, Chamomile (both Roman and German), Clary Sage, Clove, Cypress, Eucalyptus, Geranium, Lavender, Patchouli, Peppermint, Rosemary, Tea Tree, and Yarrow. Refer to the "Essential Oil Chart" for contraindications, warnings, or cautions about using essential oils.

It seems that every Christmas season, my fiancé somehow gets hurt when retrieving the ornaments and lights from the attic. One year it was a sprained ankle, another year an inflamed muscle, and the most significant was a broken foot. For someone who is so coordinated, I have to wonder is he trying to tell me something?

At the first signs of inflammation to a muscle or joint, use the Inflammation Relief blend to ease the pain and lessen swelling. However, keep in mind that pain reminds you not to overdo or shorten the healing process, so use this blend just enough to relieve the significant pain.

To treat bruises, muscle aches, or sprains anywhere on your body, apply the essential oil blends in a straight upward motion; see the "Aches & Pains" section for details.

Inflammation Relief

10 drops Chamomile

5 drops Clove

8 drops Cypress

8 drops Geranium

8 drops Lavender

> Mix all the oils together in a dark glass container. For the first 48 hours, apply a cold compress to the inflamed area as often as possible, up to 3 times per hour. Place 3 drops of the blend onto the cold wet cloth prior to each application. Keep the compress on the affected area until the cloth reaches room temperature.

> After 48 hours, add the remainder of the essential oils to 2 ounces of base lotion or 2 tablespoons carrier oil (any oil listed in the "Carrier Oils" chapter). Apply a small amount of the blend to the inflamed area and the areas immediately above and below the inflammation. Apply the blend 4 to 6 times a day for the first 3 – 5 days until the inflammation subsides.

When the pain has eased, you may want to switch to the Inflammation Soother blend. Eucalyptus, which is one ingredient of this blend, promotes the health of red and white blood cells thus facilitating healing. This blend also contains pain-relieving oils.

Inflammation Soother

10 drops Chamomile

5 drops Eucalyptus

3 drops Lavender

7 drops Peppermint

5 drops Rosemary

> Mix essential oils in 2 tablespoons of carrier oil (any oil listed in the "Carrier Oils" chapter). Massage the inflamed area. You can expect relief within 3 - 5 days.

While a lot of people don't think of sunburn as a form of inflammation, it is. When my family is on vacation, we mix the Inflammation Soother recipe in 1 cup of lukewarm water as a soothing spritzer for tender skin. It smells great and is cooling and calming at the same time.

Insects and Their Bites

"Fools rush in where angels fear to tread."

Alexander Pope

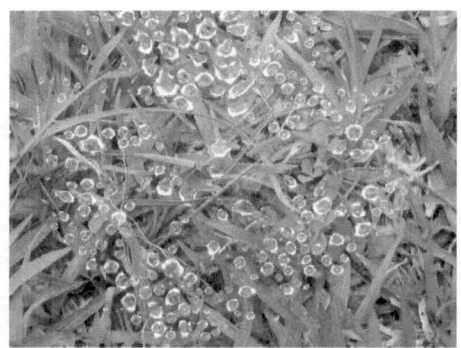

And fools we are if we rush into summer without protection from insects and their bites. You can use aromatherapy to repel insects and to relieve and heal their bites.

Mosquitoes are found in every region of the world except those frozen places such as the North Pole and Antarctica. They breed in standing water — freshwater (even if heavily polluted), saltwater marshes, and even water found in discarded containers and old tires.

Both male and female mosquitoes feed on nectar from flowers or fruit, but only female mosquitoes bite. The females require a blood meal every three to four days for the protein necessary to produce eggs. Mosquitoes bite indoors as well as outdoors so you need to prevent mosquitoes from getting inside your home and eliminate those that might already be there.

The same personal protection measures that you use against mosquitoes will also protect you against ticks and biting flies — insects that transmit Lyme disease and several other infectious diseases.

You will want to avoid mosquitoes and biting flies for another reason - insect bites, even without the risk of disease, can make you miserable. Bites usually cause localized swelling and itching, and certain bites, such as from black flies, are very painful. And, scratching those bites can cause secondary infections.

Some folksy remedies you can try are a slice of raw onion applied to a sting or meat tenderizer, which contains papain, an enzyme that breaks down the protein that makes up insect stings. To repel those flying and stinging insects burn citronella candles.

Seek medical assistance if you experience any of the following signs or symptoms:

- Difficulty breathing

- Swelling of your lips or throat

- Faintness

- Confusion

- Rapid heartbeat

- Hives

- Nausea, cramps and vomiting

You also want to see your doctor if you experience any of the less severe reactions, such as mild nausea and intestinal cramps, diarrhea, or swelling larger than 2 inches in diameter at the site.

Essential Oil Blends

It's interesting that some of the best essential oils for repelling insects are also useful for relieving the itch and pain from their bites: Chamomile, Citronella, Eucalyptus, Lavender, Lemongrass, Peppermint, Rosemary, Tea Tree, and Thyme. Refer to the "Essential Oil Chart" for contraindications, warnings, or cautions about using essential oils.

Place one drop of Lavender on a cotton swab and dab the bite – this is one of the best emergency actions you can take after a bite. Your children will appreciate that it does not sting.

Bugs Away

8 drops Eucalyptus

8 drops Lavender

8 drops Rosemary

8 drops Tea Tree

> Mix the above essential oils together. Use in any of the following ways:

> Add the oils to 2 ounces of Witch Hazel and 8 ounces of water in a spray bottle. Spray your surroundings and your skin.

> Add the oils to 5 teaspoons of olive oil. Rub this oil mixture onto your skin, especially on your pulse points on neck, wrists, and ankles, which seem to attract such critters.

You might like the light fresh aroma of this blend as an air freshener as well. *When you go out amongst the nasty little creatures, it helps to wear light colored long sleeved shirts and long pants — gives them less of a target.*

Insect Repellent

8 drops Eucalyptus

8 drops Lavender

6 drops Lemongrass

6 drops Peppermint

8 drops Rosemary

8 drops Tea Tree

> Add all of the oils together. Use in any of the following ways:
>
> Add the oils to 6 ounces of water in a spray bottle. Spray your surroundings and your skin.
>
> Add the oils to 4 ounces of base lotion or 4 tablespoons of carrier oil (any oil listed in the "Carrier Oils" chapter). Rub this oil mixture onto your skin, especially on your pulse points on neck, wrists, and ankles.
>
> Apply this insect repellent every time you are going to be in around the critters. Be careful when applying around the eyes.

Prepare the essential oil portion of the following blends at the beginning of your buggy season. That way, when the bugs bite — and they will, you don't have to take the time to mix the oils to get relief from the itch.

Don't Bug Me

12 drops Eucalyptus

24 drops Lavender

12 drops Peppermint

12 drops Rosemary

> Mix all the oils together in a dark glass container. Use in either of the following ways:
>
> Put 25 drops of the blended oils in 8 ounces of water in a spray bottle. Spray your insect bites with this blend.
>
> Add 35 drops of the essential oils to 4 ounces of base lotion or 4 tablespoons of carrier oil (any oil listed in the "Carrier Oils" chapter). Apply a small amount of the blend to the affected area 4 to 6 times a day until the bite heals. You can expect relief within 1 - 3 days.

If the insect bite has gotten a bit out of control, use the Insect Bites Relief blend because the Chamomile essential oil has a natural anti-inflammatory action that can reduce the swelling. In addition, Thyme has terrific antiseptic and antibacterial properties to keep the area from becoming infected.

Insect Bites Relief

12 drops Chamomile

24 drops Lavender

12 drops Peppermint

12 drops Thyme

> Mix all the oils together in a dark glass container. Use in either of the following ways:
>
> Put 25 drops of the blended oils in 8 ounces of water in a spray bottle. Spray your insect bites with this blend.
>
> Add 35 drops of the essential oils to 4 ounces of base lotion or 4 tablespoons of carrier oil (any oil listed in the "Carrier Oils" chapter). Apply a small amount of the blend to the affected area 4 to 6 times a day until the bite heals. You can expect relief within 1 - 3 days.

When I was a little girl, I was a magnet for insects. With tears in my eyes, skin torn from scratching, and a quivering lower lip, I would run to Mom. She would always give me hugs and say, "You can't be angry at the bugs, you have such sweet meat." Unfortunately, I passed on the sweet meat thing to my daughter, but fortunately, I also give her the motherly loving as well.

Big Relief for Little Kids

Note: This blend is safe enough to use on children as young as 18 months.

4 drops Chamomile

6 drops Eucalyptus

6 drops Lavender

Blend the oils and use them in any of the following ways:

Using a cotton swab, apply the blend to the bite.

Add the oils to a basin of water for washing the affected skin.

Add the oils to 2 tablespoons of cider vinegar, which you can dab onto the bites with a cotton ball. This may sting, but it is antiseptic as well.

Poison Ivy and Itching

*"I have a simple philosophy. Fill what's empty. Empty what's full.
And scratch what itches."*

Alice Roosevelt Longworth

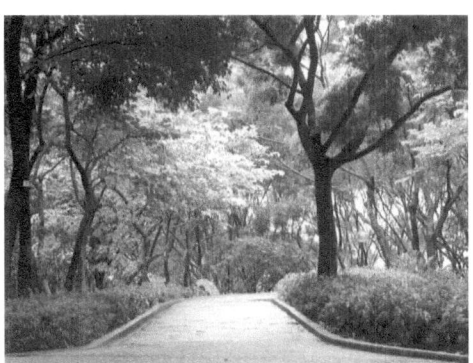

While Ms. Longworth has a good philosophy, when it comes to
scratching the itch of poison ivy, I suggest essential oils instead.
The first time you ever get poison ivy, you might not know what you
have, but you sure do itch. The second time you get poison ivy you
know exactly what it is. Gone are the questions you had the first
time. It's a good idea to learn what it looks like before you wander
out into the great outdoors. Don't be like the young woman who,
so thrilled to at last own her own home, attacked the green weeds
covering her stone wall – yes, poison ivy — wearing only shorts and
a T shirt.

One of the interesting things about plant poisoning (including poison ivy, poison oak, and poison sumac) is that the source of the poison is oil from the bruised parts of the plant. You can get this contact rash from either direct contact with the plant or through indirect contact, such as petting an animal that has rubbed against the bruised part of the plant.

You'll know when you have plant poisoning because of the itching, burning, redness, blisters, and swelling of the skin. The most important thing you can do is to remove as much of the plant oil as possible, so wash the area immediately with soap and COLD WATER. Warm or hot water will expand your pores making you that much more susceptible to the rash.

To help with the itching you can also try an antihistamine cream or take an antihistamine (such as Benadryl) to relieve some of the itching. Many people find that a tepid bath with oatmeal or in peppermint tea can also calm the skin.

Poison ivy is highly catagious so you want to avoid contact with other people and avoid scratching the itching site and then touching another part of your body, expecially around your eyes. You should contact your doctor if you have the rash around your eyes or genital areas; if the rash hasn't lessened within 5 to 7 days; or if you have any distress symptoms such as shortness of breath or high fever.

Essential Oil Blends

The best essential oils to relieve itching are Chamomile, Eucalyptus, Geranium, Lavender, Peppermint, and Tea Tree. Refer to the "Essential Oil Chart" for contraindications, warnings, or cautions about using essential oils.

My family rescues Chesapeake Bay Retrievers and we have a nice backyard in which these puppies can frolic and play. However, there is a wooded area that contains poison ivy and other plants that like to grab us. I use the Poison Ivy Relief blend on the dogs. It seems to put a nice little barrier on their fur to prevent poison ivy, which is good for them and good for my daughter who is always hugging and petting them.

Note: Be sure to reduce the number of essential oils to half when applying to a pet.

When you first get poison ivy, the thing you care about most is getting rid of the itch. Every essential oil in the Poison Ivy Relief blend contains natural chemicals to help reduce the itch. Also included are oils that soothe your skin. This is the best blend to use right from the start.

Poison Ivy Relief

15 drops Chamomile

15 drops Eucalyptus

8 drops Lemongrass

12 drops Peppermint

> Mix all the oils together in a dark glass container. Use in either of the following ways:
>
> Put 20 drops of the blended oils in 8 ounces of water in a spray bottle. When you get poison ivy, spray the area with this blend.
>
> Add 30 drops of the essential oils to 4 ounces of base lotion or 4 tablespoons of sweet almond oil. Using a cotton ball, apply a small amount of the blend to the affected area 4 to 6 times a day until the poison ivy subsides. You can expect relief within 3 - 5 days.

I formulated the Poison Ivy Soother for two reasons. Once the horrible itchiness from poison ivy has been reduced, you want to do as much as you can to heal the damaged skin. The other reason is that this blend is safe enough to use on children (3 years and older) and if you are pregnant.

Poison Ivy Soother

5 drops Chamomile

2 drops Geranium

5 drops Lavender

5 drops Tea Tree

> Mix the above oils together. Use in one of the following ways:
>
> Add the oils to 1 cup of water. Spray this blend on the affected areas. Allow it to dry naturally.
>
> To relieve a large area of skin, you might like a bath. Add the oils to 1 cup of dry oatmeal and pulverize the oats into a powder in your blender. Add about 1/4 cup of this mixture to a tepid bath. Soak until you feel better.

Calm and Heal is the best of both worlds; it contains some essential oils to reduce the itch and others to heal damaged skin.

Calm and Heal

10 drops Chamomile

8 drops Eucalyptus

8 drops Geranium

8 drops Peppermint

> You can make a body splash or a body oil.
>
> Add all of the essential oils to 2 tablespoons of base oil, such as vegetable oil or sweet almond oil. Shake well and dab on the affected area 4 to 6 times daily until the itching ceases.
>
> To make a body splash, add all of the essential oils to 8 ounces of water or peppermint tea in a spray bottle. Spritz (3 – 5 squirts) the affected area 4 to 6 times daily until the itching subsides. You can expect relief within 1 - 3 days.

When much of the damage of poison ivy has been repaired, use On the Mend to continue to nurture your skin until you are back to normal, maybe even better.

On the Mend

10 drops Chamomile

8 drops Eucalyptus

8 drops Lavender

8 drops Patchouli

> You can make a body splash or a body oil.
>
> To make a body splash, add all of the essential oils to 8 ounces of water or peppermint tea in a spray bottle. Spritz (3 – 5 squirts) the affected area 4 to 6 times daily until the itching subsides. You can expect relief within 1 – 3 days.
>
> Add all of the essential oils to 2 tablespoons of sweet almond oil. Shake well and dab on the affected area 4 to 6 times daily until the itching stops.

Sunburn

"Mad dogs and Englishmen go out in the mid-day sun."

Noel Coward

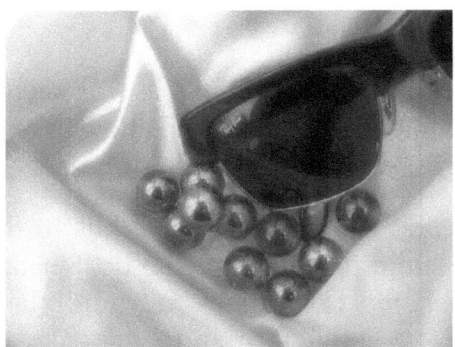

Last summer Pete, with his fair English coloring, got badly sun-burned the first time he went to the beach. Penny, also known as the Bronze Goddess, has a golden tan the entire summer. She claims she never gets a sunburn, thus doesn't have to take care, but at 40 she has skin that looks at least 10 years older.

Oh, that tantalizing sun, what could it hurt? But too much time spent in the sun today can hurt you by evening. Too much time continually spent in the sun can make you look much older before your time. And that is really the least of its evil action on your skin.

Sunburn is caused by exposure to the ultraviolet (UV) rays of the sun. Fair-skinned people are most susceptible to sunburn. People trying to get a tan too quickly in strong sunlight are also understandably vulnerable to sunburn.

Repeated sun exposure and sunburns can prematurely age the skin, causing yellowish, wrinkled skin. Overexposure, especially a serious burn in childhood, can increase the risk of skin cancer. Sunburn causes skin to turn red and blister just like any other burn. Several days later, the dead skin cells peel off, itching and flaking as they go. In severe cases, the burn may include sunstroke with vomiting and fever.

The best way to avoid sunburn is to avoid overexposure to the sun and to use sunscreen. Limit your sun time during peak "burn" hours, reapply sunscreen often, and use waterproof sunscreen when swimming or boating.

Once you have a sunburn, you have to treat the symptoms: pain, burning, and damaged skin. In addition to essential oils, you can also use vitamin C, topical creams, aloe vera gel, oatmeal baths, and cool compresses to treat the symptoms of sunburn.

Contact your doctor if your sunburn shows a sign of infection (blister filled with greenish/brownish fluid) or if the burn is on a sensitive part of your body.

Essential Oil Blends

The best essential oils for healing and relieving sunburn are Carrot, Chamomile, Clary Sage, Frankincense, Geranium, Lavender, and Rosemary. Refer to the "Essential Oil Chart" for contraindications, warnings, or cautions about using essential oils.

The following blend is safe and gentle enough for children and pregnant women, yet effective enough for tough-skinned grownups.

You can repeat it as often as you want. Use room-temperature water so you don't shock your sunburned skin.

My body is a magnet for the sun, so if I miss covering up even one small spot, I will burn. Of course, it is always in some uncomfortable spot like behind my knees.

Sunburn Stuff for Kids

3 drops Chamomile

3 drops Lavender

> Add the essential oils to 4 ounces room temperature water. Put into a spray bottle. Shake and spray. This is very soothing, and you don't have to touch the skin with a lotion.

The following blend is very cooling as well as healing to the burn.

Sunburn Pain Remedy

8 drops Lavender

4 drops Peppermint

> Mix the essential oils in 8 ounces of water. Put into a spray bottle. The water can be any temperature that is comfortable for you.

This blend is from my first aromatherapy book. It is a gentle and healing blend. *If you ever saw me at the beach, you would be hysterical. Between the wide-brimmed hats and the full-body cover-ups, you'd wonder why I even bother to show up.*

Apres Soleil Oil

5 drops Chamomile

2 drops Geranium

10 drops Lavender

> Mix the essential oils in 2 ounces of Sweet Almond oil and 2 ounces of Olive oil. Place in a plastic container. Gently rub onto your sunburned parts. You can also use 1 tablespoon of this oil as a bath oil.

Specialty Concerns

Are essential oils good for just about everything?

No conventional medication or alternative therapy is good unless you use them as suggested by a professional. One of the wonderful things about essential oils is that they work so well along with other traditional and complimentary treatments. I always tell my clients that the first step in their treatment is to go to a physician to get a diagnosis for their ailment. The doctor is also able to provide information about the ailment, and suggest methods for treating it. If you then decide to explore options, be sure to get additional information from trained and competent practitioners. You are ultimately responsible for your own health. Take the time to do your research, explore your choices, and then stick with a plan that makes sense to you.

The remainder of this section deals with:

- Athlete's Foot

- Cellulite

- Colic

- Diaper Rash

- Insomnia

- Premenstrual Syndrome and Cramps

Athlete's Foot

"No athlete is crowned, but in the sweat of his brow."

St. Jerome

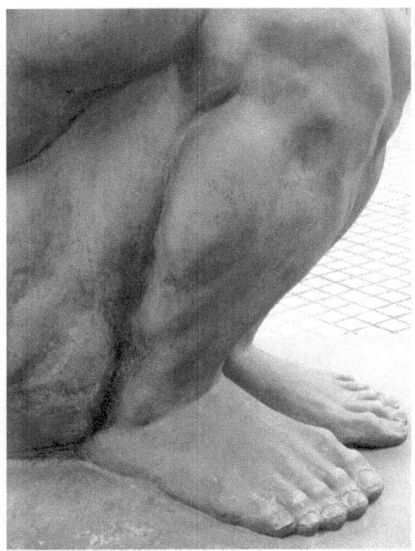

It's not the sweat of the brow that we are dealing with here, but the opposite end of the body. If you've ever been diagnosed with Athlete's foot, you don't even need to read the characteristics — you could write them for me. Itching, burning, fat feeling feet! There is nothing you wouldn't do to alleviate the symptoms or avoid catching this fungus again.

The American Podiatric Medical Association describes Athlete's Foot as a skin disease caused by a fungus, usually occurring between the toes. The fungus most commonly attacks the feet because shoes create a warm, dark, and humid environment, which encourages fungus growth.

Symptoms of athlete's foot include: dry, itchy, scaly skin, inflammation, blisters, and possibly pain, swelling, and burning. Because the fungus can live for long periods of time and is highly contagious, if you scratch the infection and then touch yourself elsewhere, you can spread it to other parts of your body, notably the groin and underarms. While athlete's foot is a common skin condition, it seems to affect teenage and adult males the most.

To help prevent athlete's foot:

- Wash your feet daily with soap and water. Soaking them in a weak apple vinegar rinse or baking soda in water will soothe and help keep the fungus discouraged. You don't want to mix the vinegar and baking soda, however, because that will make a messy chemical reaction.

- Dry your feet thoroughly (a hair dryer set to low can be helpful to dry between your toes) and keep them as dry as possible. Applying powder may also help. You can try cornstarch or powders that have cooling or soothing ingredients like chamomile or aloe vera.

- Change your shoes and socks regularly. Wear socks made of natural fibers like cotton to let your feet breath. Polyester socks will keep your feet sitting in their own perspiration. Don't wear the same shoes day after day; alternate your shoes.

- Don't walk barefoot in places where athlete's foot fungus thrives: locker room showers and pool areas. Wear rubber flip-flops to protect your feet.

Essential Oil Blends

The best essential oils for feet and fungal issues are Cypress, Eucalyptus, Geranium, Lavender, Lemon, Sage, Tea Tree, and Thyme. Refer to the "Essential Oil Chart" for contraindications, warnings, or cautions about using essential oils.

The Athlete's Foot Treatment works with cases of full-blown fungal infection along with the uncomfortable itching and damage to your skin. This is a potent blend, designed for teens and adults, which should relieve your symptoms within 5 – 7 days if used as directed.

Athlete's Foot Treatment

12 drops Geranium

20 drops Lavender

16 drops Patchouli

12 drops Rosemary

12 drops Tea Tree

16 drops Thyme

> Mix all the oils together in a dark glass container. For the first 3 days, soak your feet at least once a day. Put 12 drops of the essential oil blend in a bucket (a plastic dishpan is the perfect size – of course you would want one dedicated to your feet, not one you have to share with the dishes) of room temperature water. Soak your feet for about 20 minutes and then dry thoroughly.

> Make a lotion by adding 22 drops of the essential oil blend to 2 ounces of base lotion or 2 tablespoons of carrier oil (any oil listed in the "Carrier Oils" chapter). Apply a small amount of the blend to the affected area. If you find the oil base makes a blend that is too slick feeling for your preferences, use the lotion or aloe vera gel as your carrier.

> Add the remaining essential oil blend to 8 ounces of water and spray your feet 4 to 6 times daily until the fungus is gone. You can expect improvement within 5 – 7 days.

For younger athletes, use the Athlete's Foot Prevention blend on a regular basis. This blend is safe enough for children to use. It is a wonderful blend, with a sporty scent, that should be a part of any athlete's gym bag.

This blend is in my daughter's gym bag, not only because it prevents athlete's foot, but also because the antibacterial and anti-fungal properties of these oils help keep cold germs at bay. The feet are a great place to apply essential oils because each time you walk, the oils pump through the skin into your bloodstream.

Athlete's Foot Prevention

20 drops Lavender

20 drops Lemon

20 drops Tea Tree

16 drops Thyme

> Mix all the oils together in a dark glass container. For the first 3 days, soak your feet at least once a day. Put 10 drops of the combined essential oil blend in a bucket of room temperature water. Soak your feet for about 20 minutes, and then dry thoroughly.
>
> Make a lotion by adding 22 drops of the essential oil blend to 2 ounces of base lotion or 2 tablespoons of carrier oil (any oil listed in the "Carrier Oils" chapter). Apply a small amount of the blend to the affected area. If you find the oil base makes a blend that is too slick feeling for your preferences, use the lotion or aloe vera gel as your carrier.
>
> Add the remaining essential oil blend to 8 ounces of water and spray your feet 4 to 6 times daily until the fungus is gone. You can expect improvement within 5 – 7 days.

If you have the luxury of soaking your feet, get the most from the footbath by using the Athlete's Foot Soak blend.

Athlete's Foot Soak

10 drops Lavender

10 drops Tea Tree

> Mix oils together. Put 5 drops of the blend in a quart of water. Add one cup of salt (regular table salt or Epsom salt) and soak your feet for a good twenty minutes. You might find that this soothing bath soak is enough to take care of your itching. Try it for three days in a row. If you find that you need more help in combating this ailment, go on to the next recipe.

Some athlete's foot sufferers also have chronic skin damage. You have to go the extra mile (get it?) to keep your feet in the best condition. After using the Athlete's Foot Massage, lift your feet and relax while letting your skin absorb the carrier and essential oils. If necessary, put on cotton socks before going to bed.

Athlete's Foot Massage

6 drops Lavender

3 drops Lemon

12 drops Tea Tree

> Mix oils together. The recommended carrier oil for this massage is a combination of Borage Seed oil, Evening Primrose oil and vitamin E (available in most health food stores).

> Add the essential oils to 2 tablespoons of the carrier oil combination and massage your feet daily after soaking your feet in the Athlete's Foot Soak blend.

A natural, essential oil foot powder is a simple and effective way to keep your feet free of odor, soothed, and healthy.

Foot Powder

20 drops Lavender

20 drops Peppermint

12 drops Rosemary

16 drops Thyme

> Mix all the essential oils together and add to several teaspoons of cornstarch. This is easiest in a rounded bowl. With a spoon, mix the essential oils into the cornstarch until they are all absorbed and the cornstarch is once again in powder form. Then add this to the 1 cup of cornstarch and mix thoroughly. Store in an air tight container. A large plastic salt shaker is ideal because you can shake the powder out, yet seal it up again.

> With this recipe, use the essential oils listed in this blend, or experiment a bit to make your foot powder from a combination of essential oils mentioned at the beginning of this section.

To complement the solutions to fungal problems of the feet, treat your tootsies to a refreshing foot odor spray. Carry the spray in your gym bag so you can apply a soothing spritz to your feet and spray inside your sports shoes.

Foot Odor Spray

5 drops Lavender

5 drops Peppermint

5 drops Rosemary

5 drops Tea Tree

> Add all oils to 16 ounces of water. Use a spray bottle to give your feet a refreshing lift and deter the odors often associated with foot problems.

Cellulite

"If you could choose one characteristic that would get you through life, choose a sense of humor."

Jennifer Jones

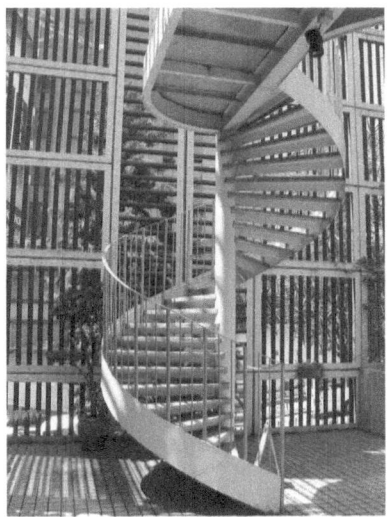

If we could choose one physical trait to avoid in life, it would be cellulite — that nasty grapefruit-looking flesh that can creep up on anyone! It doesn't care about your age, your exercise regime, or your vanity. Unfortunately there are no quick cures for cellulite. You have to work at eradicating it. The blends in this chapter should help.

Cellulite is a common term used to describe superficial pockets of trapped fat, which cause uneven, wrinkled, dimply skin. Cellulite can be found on the thighs, buttocks, and abdomen in about 90% of post-adolescent women. It is rarely seen in men (yet another thing we can love about them). Contrary to popular belief, cellulite is not related to obesity, since it occurs in overweight, normal, and thin women. It is actually formed when the connective tissues beneath the skin that shapes the fat becomes weak and deformed.

There are several theories about what causes cellulite including poor elimination of toxins, hormones that regulate fat storage, and metabolism in the fat layer. Others suggest that the primary cause of cellulite is poor blood and lymph circulation, not exercise and diet.

Exercise is a great way to burn fat and improve circulation. Although exercise will not cure cellulite, when used together with detoxification and improved circulation of the affected areas, it can reduce the appearance of cellulite. Another way to improve circulation is with massage and friction rubs.

Nicole Ronsard, the author of "Cellulite: Those Lumps, Bumps and Bulges You Couldn't Lose Before" has several excellent books out on the subject. You should check them out for an understanding of how your lifestyle may contribute to cellulite. She will also give you some helpful information to create a plan to deal with it.

One of the best things you can do for yourself right away is drink water. Start right now!

Essential Oil Blends

The best essential oils for treating cellulite are Basil, Cypress, Fennel, Geranium, Grapefruit, Juniper, Lavender, Lemon, Orange, Rosemary, and Thyme. Refer to the "Essential Oil Chart" for contraindications, warnings, or cautions about using essential oils.

The key to success with cellulite is to aggressively massage the affected area for a full minute twice daily, every single day. Don't miss a single day. You must be prepared to commit to a twice daily workout on your cellulite areas for at least 3 months. Remember it took a long time for you to acquire that cellulite. It will take a while to improve it.

Before you use the cellulite treatments, take a warm shower and use a loofah, brush or friction rub (one with pumice or ground almonds in it is good). This gets the circulation revved up and the pores open to accept the aromatherapy treatment.

If you want some change after using the following blends, experiment a bit with the essential oils listed at the beginning of this section. Replace one or two essential oils in the following blend recipes with similar essential oils from the list. For example, you could replace Lemon with Orange.

Deluxe Cellulite Treatment

6 drops Cypress

6 drops Fennel

8 drops Grapefruit

4 drops Juniper

4 drops Lemon

4 drops Rosemary

> You can put all of the essential oils in either 2 ounces of base lotion or 2 tablespoons of carrier oil (any oil listed in the "Carrier Oils" chapter)

> Aggressively massage a small amount of the blend on the affected area for a full minute twice daily, every single day.

At first, it feels like your arms may fall off before you complete the full minute, but keep working at it. Now, I can go for about 4 minutes of aggressive massage without breaking a sweat!

Another series of essential oils that are very effective in treating cellulite have been used in Europe for many years and are included in the European Cellulite Treatment.

European Cellulite Treatment

10 drops Basil

8 drops Fennel

10 drops Grapefruit

14 drops Juniper

10 drops Lemon

6 drops Tangerine

> You can put all of the essential oils in either 2 ounces of base lotion or 2 tablespoons of carrier oil (any oil listed in the "Carrier Oils" chapter)

> Aggressively massage a small amount of the blend on the affected area for a full minute twice daily, every single day.

You know that loose skin that hangs down from your arm, so that when you wave, that skin is still flapping well after the wave is over? Well, after using this blend for three months, and exercising those arms by aggressively massaging twice daily, I noticed that the skin tightened up. So I got two benefits — no cellulite and no flabby arms – yeah!

Colic

"Diaper backward spells repaid. Think about it."

Marshall McLuhan

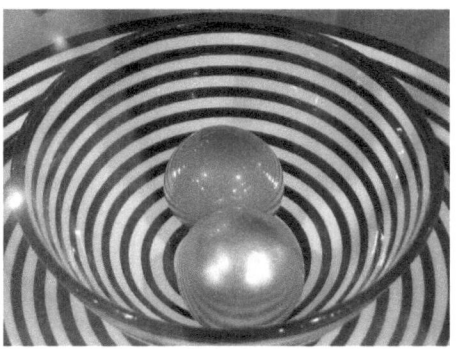

Diaper spelled backwards spells repaid – I laugh each time I read that line. Humor is a wonderful strategy to help us get through some of the tension and stress that we have in our everyday lives. However, when there is a physical ailment of unknown origin that is affecting your helpless newborn – and you as well, a good joke just doesn't seem to cut it. Fortunately, aromatherapy can help.

There are many myths about the causes and cure of colic, but there is no concrete evidence. What we do know is that about 25% of all children born in the United States will suffer with colic, which is described as severe abdominal pain. The other thing we know is that both the parents and the child suffer. If your baby has a constant and piercing cry, is red-faced, has a hard tummy, with legs drawn up, and coldness in the hands and feet; then your little one is suffering from colic.

The good news, if there is any, is that colic doesn't last forever, that colicky babies are often in great health, and are otherwise very happy.

So what can you do? While no scientific evidence supports a cure, some things that parents believe have helped are playing soft music, patting your baby's back, speaking in a soothing voice, white noise, walking, rocking, humming, singing, and burping — all those loving things we do for our children anyway.

Essential Oil Blends

Essential oils that assist in treating colic are: Carrot, Chamomile (both Roman and German), Clary Sage, Clove, Dill, Fennel, Ginger, Lavender, Marjoram, Peppermint, Parsley, Black Pepper, and Rosemary. Refer to the "Essential Oil Chart" for contraindications, warnings, or cautions about using essential oils.

A client came to me with a newborn suffering from colic and an 18-month old with an ear infection. In addition to give her the blends for colic and earaches, I made a soothing, stress relief blend for her.

The Colic Relief contains oils that are safe to use on infants.

Colic Relief

5 drops Chamomile

5 drops Lavender

5 drops Geranium

> Add all essential oils to 4 ounces of base lotion or 4 tablespoons of carrier oil (any oil listed in the "Carrier Oils" chapter). **Gently** apply a small amount of the blend to your baby's abdomen and to the lower back around the kidney area in soft, circular motions. Apply the blend 4 to 6 times a day until the pain subsides. You can expect relief within 3 – 5 days.

> Of course, soothing lullabies, gentle hugs, and a ton of patience are also required.

Even if you have only Chamomile, you can still get some relief from colic.

Colic Soother

1 drop Chamomile

> Put one drop of Chamomile essential oil in your palm. Pour about one teaspoon of Olive Oil into your palm. Rub your palms together, warming the oil mixture and spreading it around your palms. Gently rub some of this on your baby's belly. Don't rush. Cover the baby's belly with an undershirt or a soft blanket to keep in the warmth. You can expect relief within 3 – 5 days.

I know that 3 – 5 days sounds like a terribly long time for a parent who is sleep-deprived and cranky, so be sure to start this blend at the first sign of colic. Keep in mind that Chamomile is very soothing for infants, so when in doubt, make this blend and let your baby enjoy a gentle massage.

Diaper Rash

"There are two ways of meeting difficulties. You alter the difficulties or you alter yourself to meet them."

Phyliss Bottome

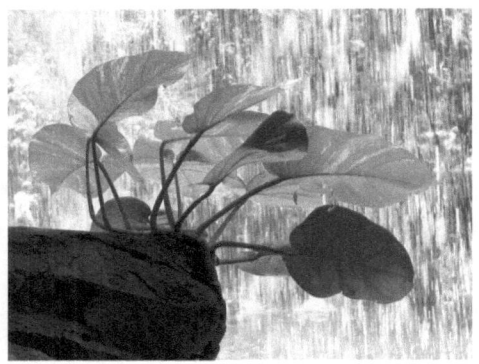

I had to pick this quote because of the woman's last name. Your poor baby has a diaper rash. You've been vigilant in checking for wetness and changing frequently. But there it is and you can tell it hurts. It hurts you almost as much as it hurts your baby. As Ms. Bottome says you can alter the difficulty and, in this case, essential oils can provide relief from diaper rash.

Diaper rash is one of the few skin disorders for which the cause is known — irritants and wetness trapped in a diaper. Other factors that contribute to diaper rash are changes in your baby's formula, beginning solid foods, teething, or taking an antibiotic. An untreated diaper rash causes painful breaks in the skin that can become deeper and spread out to cover a larger area.

No formal diagnosis is required as diaper rash is easy to spot because of the location of the slightly red skin of the diaper area. More severe cases can also include small pimples or blisters in addition to redness. The tender baby skin becomes uncomfortable.

Treat diaper rash at the first sign of redness by cleaning the skin gently but thoroughly and allowing the diaper area to dry completely. Be sure to do this every time you change your baby, and check that diaper often.

Essential Oil Blends

The best essential oils for baby's skin are Chamomile, Cypress, Geranium, Lavender, Patchouli, and Yarrow. Refer to the "Essential Oil Chart" for contraindications, warnings, or cautions about using essential oils.

With the thick lotion that many commercial diaper rash treatments provide, it seems like you need a chisel to get the lotion off your baby's sensitive skin. With the essential oil blends mixed in a soothing oil or lotion, you can have the same effective relief with a much more gentle touch.

During the day, the Diaper Rash Relief blend is very helpful. The light fragrance is a joy to a baby's nose while the natural ingredients treat their sensitive diaper area.

Diaper Rash Relief

10 drops Lavender

10 drops Yarrow

> Add all of the essential oils to 2 ounces of base lotion or 2 tablespoons of carrier oil (any oil listed in the "Carrier Oils" chapter). Apply a small amount of the blend to the cute little tooshie area every time you change your baby. You can expect relief within 3 – 5 days.

I always used the Diaper Rash Treatment at night because in addition to providing a safe and effective way to get rid of diaper rash, the Chamomile in this blend was a gentle and mild sedative that helped my little girl sleep.

Diaper Rash Treatment

2 drop Chamomile

6 drops Geranium

4 drops Lavender

> Clean the diaper area with warm water to which you have added a drop of Chamomile. Use a soft 100% cotton towel or cloth.
>
> Mix the essential oils together. You can use this blend in any of the following ways:
>
> Add the oils to 2 tablespoons Almond oil and massage baby's diaper area to lessen diaper rash.
>
> Use 1 drop of the blend in a pleasant bath.
>
> For a persistent diaper rash, combine this blend with water instead of the base oil, spritz the child's diaper area, and then sprinkle on cornstarch.
>
> If diaper rash has caused your child to be fretful and uncomfortable, you can make a double batch of this blend and use it to give your child a relaxing and soothing massage. Don't forget to use firm but gentle strokes, and make the experience even more memorable with a calming lullaby.

Keeping your baby's diaper area clean, aerated, and smooth helps prevent diaper rash. The Diaper Rash Prevention blend is great for children over 18 months old.

Diaper Rash Prevention

4 drops Cypress

10 drops Lavender

4 drops Patchouli

> Add all of the essential oils to 2 ounces of base lotion or 2 tablespoons of carrier oil (any oil listed in the "Carrier Oils" chapter). Apply a small amount of the blend to the cute little tooshie area every time you change your baby. You can expect relief within 3 – 5 days.

Insomnia

"Not everything that can be counted counts, and not everything that counts can be counted."

Albert Einstein

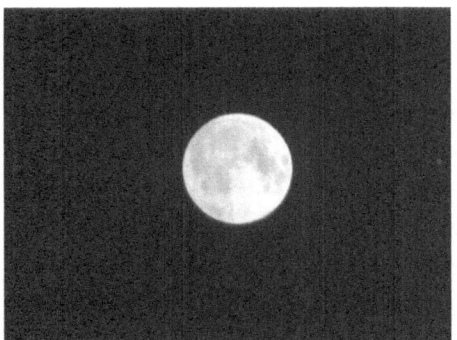

If we pondered all of the possibilities of what Einstein meant in this quotation, we could probably fall asleep faster than if we counted sheep. And, if pondering Einstein helps you get to sleep, you might just have another thing to thank Albert for.

In the hustle and bustle of today's busy world, insomnia might seem like a normal part of life, but actually, insomnia is the body's way of saying that something isn't right. The most common causes of insomnia are stress, too much caffeine, depression, change, and pain. While most people will occasionally experience insomnia, you do not want the abbreviated sleep pattern to become a habit. Once established as a habit, insomnia is harder to relieve. While insomnia is not a serious health problem, it can cause difficult days by making you feel tired, depressed, or irritable.

There are several natural strategies you can use to help relieve insomnia. Having a sleep routine is important, including going to bed and waking at the same time each day, and doing something restful just before bed such as taking a warm bath. Avoid watching television before bed — who could possibly sleep when the news was the last thing they saw? Other professionals suggest journaling to help clear your mind before bed. Having something useful but boring to think about is helpful. Every time your mind starts racing think of your boring subject instead. Also, keep the bedroom quiet and dark, and avoid caffeine and alcohol past 6:00 pm.

Exercise, a good diet, and stress-relieving activities will positively impact how you fall asleep as well as how you enjoy your days. Some of Grandma's home remedies have received scientific validity, such as a warm glass of milk and a cookie, a cup of chamomile tea, or a warm bath. We always knew we should listen to our grandmothers.

Many people who suffer from insomnia seek their doctor's assistance during the early stages of their sleep disorder. As insomnia is a symptom, not an ailment, your doctor may be able to rule out some ailments and help you more clearly define what might be causing your insomnia. Your doctor can also discuss prescribed and over-the-counter medications, supplements, and other alternatives.

Essential Oil Blends

Good essential oils for insomnia are: Cedarwood, Clary Sage, Chamomile (both German and Roman), Geranium, Lavender, Marjoram, Orange, Sandalwood, Valerian, and Vetiver. Refer to the

"Essential Oil Chart" for contraindications, warnings, or cautions about using essential oils.

With prescription and over-the-counter medication, some formulas work better for some people while others seem to give little or no relief. The same applies to the natural chemicals that we use in essential oil blends. The recipes provided here have been used by hundreds of people. The Insomnia Relief works great for many but the Insomnia Body Rub has helped when other solutions have not. Try any of these blends to find the one that works best for you.

The Insomnia Relief blend is recommended for adults. You can use this blend and take prescribed or over-the-counter medication as well. However, once you have several consecutive nights of good sleep, start weaning yourself off the synthetic products and rely on the natural solution.

Insomnia Relief

6 drops Clary Sage

6 drops Lavender

2 drops Valerian

4 drops Vetiver

> Add all of the essential oils to 8 ounces of water in a spray bottle. Before going to bed, spritz (3 – 5 squirts) your pillow, your nightgown, and your chest. After approximately 7 – 10 days, you should be getting better sleep. After 3 consecutive good nights of sleep, you can start weaning yourself by spraying only the pillow and your chest. If your sleep is just as restful, stay at this level for 2 more weeks, then you can wean to spraying just the pillow.

Note: At any time that you need extra support, go back to spraying your pillow, bed clothing, and chest.

Sweet Dreams is a great blend for children ages 6 to 18. The fragrance is pleasant and calming and the essential oils contain mild sedatives that offer a natural solution when your child is suffering from sleeplessness.

Sweet Dreams

4 drops Chamomile

4 drops Clary Sage

8 drops Lavender

4 drops Orange

> Add all of the essential oils to 8 ounces of water in a spray bottle. Before bedtime, spritz (3 – 5 squirts) your child's pillow, pajamas, and chest. After approximately 7 – 10 days, your child should be getting better sleep. After 3 consecutive good nights of sleep, you can start weaning your child by spraying only the pillow and your child's chest. If sleep is just as restful, stay at this level for 2 more weeks, then you can wean to spraying just the pillow.

Note: At any time that you need extra support, go back to spraying your pillow, bed clothing, and chest.

Go ahead and spoil yourself with the Insomnia Body Rub. This blend seems to be a particular favorite of men because of the woodsy fragrance of the Cedarwood combined with the sedative properties of all three essential oils.

Insomnia Body Rub

12 drops Cedarwood

6 drops Clary Sage

12 drops Orange

> Mix the oils and use in one of the following ways:
>
> Combine the essential oils with 2 ounces carrier oil. Use this as a body rub to *really relax* you before bedtime.
>
> Add the essentials oil blend to 2 tablespoons lotion and rub a little on your pulse points (wrist and temples) before bedtime.

Insomnia Bath blend is a favorite for woman. I'm not sure if that's because using it makes you take 20 minutes for yourself everyday, or if the feminine properties of Geranium and Clary Sage touch you to the core. Either way, relax and enjoy!

Insomnia Bath

2 drops Cedarwood

2 drops Chamomile

1 drop Clary Sage

2 drops Geranium

> Mix the essential oils in 2 ounces Hazelnut Oil, 2 ounces Milk, or ½ cup of Epsom Salts. Use the Hazelnut Oil if your skin is suffering from residual effects of a long, cold, windy winter. Use the milk for some soothing. Pour this into a tub of warm water and relax for 20 minutes.

Sleeplessness Relief for Children is very effective for toddlers and children up to the age of 12. It is safe and soothing for our young insomniacs as young as 18 months old.

Sleeplessness Relief for Children

6 drops Chamomile

8 drops Lavender

6 drops Orange

> Mix all ingredients in 8 oz of water in a spray bottle. Spray bed clothing and room air before bedtime.

The critics have spoken, "Sleep For Sure works so well it is almost addictive!" Fortunately, it is safe, natural, and non-addictive. "Sleep for Sure" was my faithful standby when I was suffering through a bout of insomnia.

Sleep For Sure

9 drops Clary Sage

6 drops Lemon

6 drops Vetiver

> Mix the essential oils in 2 tablespoons lotion. Apply to neck and wrist pulse points before going to bed.

Premenstrual Syndrome and Cramps

"It is easier to find men who will volunteer to die, than to find those who are willing to endure pain with patience."

Julius Caesar

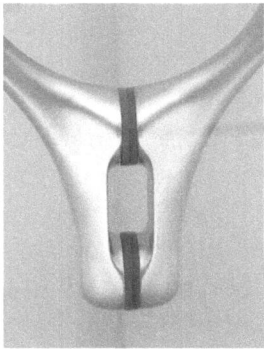

And endure pain with patience, women must. For those of us who suffer from premenstrual syndrome (PMS) or menstrual cramps, every month becomes an endurance contest with the pain, distress, odor, and bloating often associated with our cycle.

I read an article once that suggested that if we viewed our menstrual cycle as a celebration of our womanhood, we would be able to reduce the physical discomfort associated with it. Since I have a daughter on the cusp of this experience, I have been sharing that thought with her and honestly I do believe it has helped me.

PMS - If you've never had PMS then it may be difficult for you to understand the physical and emotional symptoms that millions of women experience each month about 7 to 14 days before their period. For those of you who do experience acne, bloating, constipation, crying spells, feeling irritable, tension, fatigue, anxiety, tender and swollen breasts, swollen hands or feet, there is help.

Changes in hormonal levels seem to be linked to PMS. While there is no cure for PMS, there are some things you can do to ease the symptoms. Eat a healthy diet (cut back on sugar, salt, and fats), exercise regularly (30 minutes, 4 to 6 times a week) and get a good night's sleep. In addition, cut back on caffeine and alcohol to feel less tense, depressed, and to ensure that you get a good night's sleep.

There are several vitamins, supplements, natural chemical products, over-the-counter medications, diuretics, and more that can help you during PMS. Because treatments vary, try not to get discouraged if it takes some time to find tips or strategies help.

Cramps - While some of us breeze through our menstrual cycles with little acknowledgement, others may suffer from cramp-like spasms that start in the lower abdomen, and may radiate up the spine and down the legs, or center in the lower back. Most women find the pain usually comes on a few hours before their periods start and begins to ease once the flow begins. But in a few, pain continues into the second and even the third day of their period.

To help relieve menstrual cramps, try lying down at the first sign of pain and placing a warm heating pad on your abdomen. A relaxing, warm bath may also help as can massage and exercise.

If you have unbearable pain with nausea and vomiting, you should consult a doctor who may prescribe pain-relieving medication or birth control pills to reduce the production of hormones that contribute to the pain.

Essential Oil Blends

Essential oils that assist in managing cramps and menstrual discomfort are: Basil, Carrot, Chamomile (both Roman and German), Clary Sage, Cypress, Fennel, Frankincense, Juniper, Lavender, Marjoram, Rosemary, Sage, and Yarrow. For PMS, use Bergamot, Carrot, Chamomile (both Roman and German), Geranium, Grapefruit, Lavender, Marjoram, Nutmeg, Orange, and Palma Rosa. Refer to the "Essential Oil Chart" for contraindications, warnings, or cautions about using essential oils.

You must be prepared to use a PMS blend faithfully twice daily for 3 months to achieve benefit. But for those of us who have suffered with PMS symptoms, these blends are a precious gift well worth the time.

After you achieve the desired emotional/hormonal balance (which may take 3 months or more), you can start weaning yourself. For the first two weeks, I applied the blend twice daily Monday, Wednesday, and Friday, and only once on Tuesday, Thursday, Saturday, and Sunday. When things were still fine, after about 2 weeks (just to make sure), I dropped down to once daily. After three weeks, I dropped down to every other day. Now, I use it once a week.

Note: At any time that you feel the PMS returning, start using the blend as often as you used it at your previous success level.

Since our PMS demons make take on a variety of appearances, we offer essential oil solutions customized for the particular fiend that joins you each month. Use PMS Soother for gentle, soothing relief from premenstrual symptoms.

PMS Soother

10 drops Chamomile

10 drops Geranium

10 drops Lavender

> Add all essential oils to 4 ounces of base lotion or 4 tablespoons of carrier oil (any oil listed in the "Carrier Oils" chapter) (note: oil can stain your panties, I use lotion).

> Apply a small amount of the blend in a **V** pattern starting from the top of the vaginal area, up over your hips, and down to the top of the buttocks.

PMS Relief for Tension provides a bit more tension relief.

PMS Relief for Tension

22 drops Bergamot

8 drops Geranium

15 drops Nutmeg

> Add all essential oils to 4 ounces of base lotion or 4 tablespoons of carrier oil (any oil listed in the "Carrier Oils" chapter) (note: oil can stain your panties, I use lotion).

> Apply a small amount of the blend in a **V** pattern starting from the top of the vaginal area, up over your hips, and down to the top of the buttocks.

If you are feeling like a melancholy baby during this time, PMS Uplifter offers uplifting emotional support.

PMS Uplifter

5 drops Bergamot

15 drops Clary Sage

25 drops Grapefruit

> Add all essential oils to 4 ounces of base lotion or 4 tablespoons of carrier oil (any oil listed in the "Carrier Oils" chapter) (note: oil can stain your panties, I use lotion).

> Apply a small amount of the blend in a **V** pattern starting from the top of the vaginal area, up over your hips, and down to the top of the buttocks.

If you are feeling crabby, use PMS Relief for Grumps.

PMS Relief for Grumps

15 drops Bergamot

15 drops Geranium

15 drops Orange

> Add all essential oils to 4 ounces of base lotion or 4 tablespoons of carrier oil (any oil listed in the "Carrier Oils" chapter) (note: oil can stain your panties, I use lotion).

> Apply a small amount of the blend in a **V** pattern starting from the top of the vaginal area, up over your hips, and down to the top of the buttocks.

Lighten your spirits with PMS Lifter.

PMS Lifter

15 drops Bergamot

15 drops Clary Sage

15 drops Rosemary

> Add all essential oils to 4 ounces of base lotion or 4 tablespoons of carrier oil (any oil listed in the "Carrier Oils" chapter) (note: oil can stain your panties, I use lotion).

> Apply a small amount of the blend in a **V** pattern starting from the top of the vaginal area, up over your hips, and down to the top of the buttocks.

Both Cramp Relief for Tummies and Cramp Relief for All Over offer calming, hormonally balancing and pain relieving support.

Cramp Relief for Tummies

8 drops Clary Sage

4 drops Fennel

4 drops Geranium

> Mix the essential oils in 1 tablespoon carrier oil. Massage the blend in a **V** pattern starting from the top of the vaginal area, up over your hips, and down to the top of the buttocks.

Cramp Relief for All Over

6 drops Chamomile

8 drops Fennel

8 drops Lavender

> Mix oils together and add them to 2 tablespoons vegetable oil. Massage the blend in a **V** pattern starting from the top of the vaginal area, up over your hips, and down to the top of the buttocks.

Next Steps

You know the expression, "armed and dangerous"? Well, I hope this book has armed you with information that is not dangerous and gives you more control over managing your health.

Many of my clients have suffered from the negative side effects of synthetic solutions, without receiving any relief. They've asked me, "What else can I do?"

Now you have a choice – you have Aromatherapy Answers!

Carriers

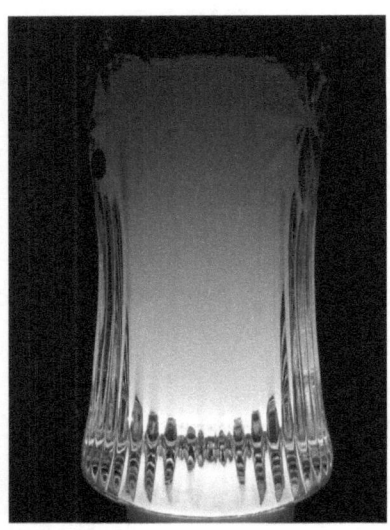

What is a carrier?

When discussing aromatherapy, a carrier is the base product you use to make blends. Most essential oils are too strong to be applied directly to the skin, some sting the skin and some burn (cinnamon comes to mind as one of the burning ones). Essential oils are also too precious to use more than you need. Using a carrier as the base for your blend allows you to get maximum coverage, dilutes the essential oils as necessary, and allows you to use only the exact amount of essential oils you need for each blend.

Some aromatherapists consider a wide variety of products to be "carriers" because the carrier product is *carrying* the essential oils safely to the body and allowing the chemical properties of the essential oils to enter the bloodstream. In light of this definition, water, shampoo, bath gels, lotions, creams, and many other products can be used as carriers.

In this book, I most frequently use carrier oils and other natural substances (aloe vera, for instance) for two reasons. First, they work very well with essential oils and do not interfere with the curative properties of the essential oils. Second, as you see in this chapter, many of these oils have their own therapeutic value.

What is a base oil?

The vegetable and seed oils presented in the recipes are generally extracted from seeds, fruits, or vegetables. They are high in fat content (thus in energy potential) and highly emollient (thus easy to spread around). Oils that are cold pressed (extracted without the use of heat or chemicals) are preferable because the cold pressing process leaves most (perhaps all) of the benefit of these natural ingredients. Base oils are composed mainly of fatty acids, proteins, minerals, and vitamins.

Note: Avoid products that are derived from petroleum products, petroleum jelly, for instance.

Other substances to use for a base

In addition to using oils, you can also use some other natural substances as a base:

Aloe vera (the juice of a plant)

Vinegar

Vodka

Milk (dairy, nut, or vegetable)

Witch Hazel

Herbal tea

Honey

Yogurt

Fruit or vegetable juice

What's the difference?

You would vary your carrier depending upon the condition of the skin, what you are adding for essential oils, and what you want as a result. For instance, you might use vinegar, vodka, or witch hazel in a skin toner for an oily skin condition. On the other hand, you would use oil, milk, or honey to add moisture to skin that is dry. Herbal teas would be chosen for the action of the herb itself. Chamomile tea, for instance, would calm the skin. The acidic action of yogurt or juices would be an aid to certain skin conditions such as acne or oily skin.

Also keep in mind that you can use a combination of the base oil and other base substances in your blend. For example, you might use a combination of evening primrose oil and aloe vera for your base carrier when formulating a blend for sunburn because the evening primrose oil is very effective for damaged skin and the aloe vera reduces dryness and irritation.

Location, location, location

For the most part you can find the recommended bases in the grocery store or in your health food store. Even oil, such as sweet almond oil, that might seem expensive when you are considering using it to cook with, is an absolute bargain when you compare it against the cost of most cosmetic skin applications. Generally a teaspoon is too much for a facial, just about right for a massage. Figure in the cost of the essential oils (which you should always add AFTER you have measured out and mixed your base combination) and you still have a healthy solution that costs just pennies.

Storage considerations

Store most oils in cool or cold places. The refrigerator is perfect for some oils. Others do well in a cool (not cold) dry dark place. Do keep in mind that some oils, olive oil is one, seem to become a sludge (not an attractive sight, I know) when they are chilled in the fridge. But a few minutes at room temperature and they resume their golden glow. The cool storage is to keep them from spoiling or turning rancid, a process in which they lose their healthful action and begin to take on an unpleasant odor. Not what you want to use when you are creating a wholesome blend.

Aloe vera, any of the milks, yogurt, and the juices should definitely be stored in the refrigerator and not kept for very long because they lose their freshness. Milk sours, yogurt becomes moldy, and juice ferments. Honey, if kept too long, crystallizes. You can reconstitute it by adding a bit of water and heating it, then stirring in the water. Heat honey gently either in a double boiler or in the microwave, adding a bit of water if necessary.

Therapeutic properties?

Vitamins, trace elements, minerals, fatty acids – most of the oils in this chapter are from living material.

About the Carrier Oils

There is a great deal of information about carrier oils, such as their plant of origin, their color, and in what products they are frequently used. Much of this information is beyond the scope of this book, but when it comes to choosing the carrier oils you want to use for the recipes in this book, there are three things you want to know:

- Does the carrier have a scent (that might interfere with a fragrance you are trying to achieve, especially in those recipes that suggest scent therapy benefits)?

- What is the best way to store the carrier so they last, especially since the essential oils have a shelf life of about 18 months?

- How well does the carrier apply to the skin?

So the following list provides you information about those three items.

Sweet Almond Oil is lightly sweet and nutty. It is oily enough to leave a residue. It is a nourishing and soothing oil that is close to the oil found naturally in the skin. Store in a well-filled (so there is little air to oxygenate it), airtight container at a cool temperature, protected from light.

Aloe Vera Gel has a light spring-like odor. It absorbs quickly, leaving no residue. It softens the skin, reducing dryness and irritation. It is very potent in healing burns, whether from heat or from the sun, and is very refreshing. Store aloe vera in an airtight container at a cool temperature, protected from light.

Apricot (Kernel) Oil is almost odorless (which is a shame, I would like it to smell like fresh apricots). It is somewhat greasy, leaving a residue. It is an excellent moisturizer for face and hands and is a nourishing addition to creams and body oils. Store this oil in a well-filled, airtight container at a cool temperature, protected from light.

Avocado Oil has a pleasant lingering nutty scent and a thick texture. A highly penetrable and spreadable oil, it leaves a non-sticky sheen on your skin, making it an excellent moisturizer. Keep cool, but do not chill. Keeps well.

Borage Oil is slightly sweet. Its texture is thin, but oily. It is rapidly absorbed by the skin, leaving no residue. It is close in composition to Evening Primrose oil. It is good for damaged skin, dermatitis, eczema, psoriasis, hair, and nails. To store, keep it in a well-filled, airtight container at a cool temperature, protected from light.

Camellia Oil has a very light fragrance. This is another oil that is readily absorbed leaving no oily residue. This oil is light and nourishing for facial blends. Store in a well-filled, airtight container at a cool temperature, protected from light.

Coconut Oil does smell like coconut. It is a thick, semi solid oil at room temperature that melts easily at body temperature. High in saturated fatty acids, it forms an easily absorbable ointment base. It lathers well, so use it in soaps and shampoos and it is recommended for scalp treatments. Because it becomes rancid if exposed to air, store in a well-filled, airtight container at a cool temperature, protected from light.

Corn Oil has a slight fragrance. It is effective for all skin types and is often used in moisturizing creams and lotions. Store in a well-filled, airtight container at a cool temperature, protected from light.

Evening Primrose Oil has only a slight fragrance. While it is oily in texture, it is absorbed quickly into the skin. This oil is effective for aging, sun-damaged skin, eczema, wounds, and dandruff. Store in a well-filled, airtight container at a cool temperature, protected from light.

Grapeseed Oil has a faintly sweet, nutty smell. Although it is absorbed quickly, grapeseed oil leaves an oily residue. With its mildly astringent properties, it is best used for acne and oily skin. While this oil keeps well, you still want to store it away from light and heat.

Hazelnut Oil is light and nutty in aroma. This oil is quickly absorbed and adds moisture to skin with no oily residue. Hazelnut oil is an excellent moisturizing base for oily skin. Another oil that keeps well, but should be stored away from light and heat.

Jojoba Oil is actually a wax, not an oil. The oil is thick but is rapidly absorbed, and leaves your skin feeling smooth. Similar to sebum, the natural oil produced by our own skin, jojoba oil is suitable for all types of skin, particularly aging skin. A very stable oil, jojoba oil should be stored in cool temperatures.

Kukui Nut Oil is lightly sweet and nutty. It is absorbed rapidly and leaves no greasy feeling. Kukui nut oil is helpful in treating eczema and dermatitis. Store in opaque, well-filled, airtight containers in cool temperature.

Macadamia Nut Oil is more sweet and nutty than some of the other nut-based oils. This thick oil is absorbed slowly and leaves an oily residue. Useful in body oils, this oil is also good for dry, mature skin. Store this oil away from light and heat.

Olive Oil does have the expected olive smell. It has a fairly thick and oily texture. Olive oil is nutritious and soothing to skin. Olive oil is also very gentle on baby's skin. Good for bath oils and ointments. Store in a well-filled, airtight container at a cool temperature, protected from light.

Peanut Oil has a faint nutty scent and a thin oily texture, which leaves a greasy film. Peanut oil is good in creams for dry skin, and arthritic and rheumatic conditions. Store in a well-filled, airtight container at a cool temperature, protected from light.

Pecan Oil has a very faint nutty scent. It absorbs into skin moderately quickly but leaves a slight oily film. This oil is fairly unstable and should be stored (for only a short period of time) in a well-filled, airtight container at a cool temperature, protected from light.

Safflower Oil has a slightly nutty scent. It has an oily texture and leaves a slightly greasy film. This oil is effective in blends for arthritic pain, bruises, and sprains. Store carefully in a cool place. This oil thickens and becomes rancid with prolonged exposure to air.

Sesame Oil has a distinctive sweet nutty scent. This oil has a somewhat greasy feeling to it. Sesame oil is excellent for rheumatic conditions, for psoriasis, dry skin, and eczema. This oil requires cool storage.

Sunflower Seed Oil has a faint sweet scent. It has a light texture that leaves skin smooth and non-greasy feeling. This oil is useful for treating bruises and dermatitis. Store in a well-filled, airtight container at a cool temperature, protected from light.

Wheat Germ Oil has a nutty scent. Thick and heavy in texture, this oil is an excellent source of vitamin E. It keeps skin soft and supple and exhibits healing qualities for cuts and wounds. Store this oil in a well-filled, airtight container at a cool temperature, protected from light.

How do you choose?

Once again, rely on yourself. The chart below suggests bases that have proven abilities for a specific problem. Once you have selected some appropriate bases based upon their therapeutic value, smell the base you are considering. Rub a bit into your skin. Does it seem pleasing? Keep in mind the health challenge you are facing. Does this base feel appropriate for that purpose? Your intuition can count here.

Chart

Therapeutic areas covered in our book	Bases
Acne	Grapeseed oil, Hazelnut oil, Jojoba oil
Aging Skin	Sweet almond oil, Apricot kernel oil, Avocado oil, Borage oil, Evening Primrose Oil, Jojoba oil, Olive oil, Wheat Germ oil
Arthritic Conditions	Peanut Oil, Safflower oil, Sesame oil
Burns	Aloe vera gel
Cellulite	Hazelnut oil
Dandruff	Evening Primrose Oil
Dry Skin	Sweet almond oil, Apricot kernel oil, Aloe vera gel, Avocado oil, Olive oil, Wheat Germ oil
Eczema	Sweet almond oil, Avocado oil, Borage oil, Evening Primrose Oil, Jojoba oil, Olive oil, Sesame oil, Wheat Germ oil
Hair	Jojoba oil
Inflammation	Sweet almond oil, Apricot kernel oil, Aloe vera gel, Hazelnut oil, Olive oil, Jojoba oil, Sunflower Seed Oil
Itching	Sweet almond oil
Nails	Borage oil
Psoriasis	Borage oil, Evening Primrose Oil, Jojoba oil, Olive oil, Sesame oil, Wheat Germ oil
Rheumatic Conditions	Olive oil, Peanut oil, Sesame oil
Sunburn	Aloe vera gel, Evening Primrose Oil

Essential Oil Chart

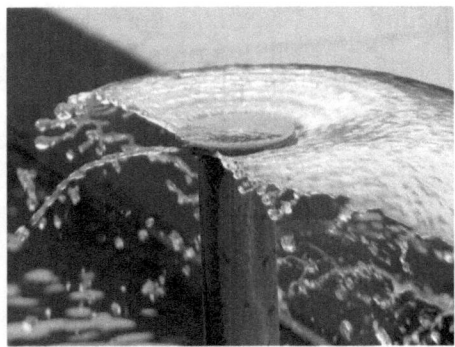

This quick reference chart provides an overview of the essential oils that are used in blends in this book.

Why should I care about the Latin name?

If you are going to buy essential oils and make your own blends, use the Latin name to make sure you are buying the proper essential oils. Some common names, such as Marjoram, may actually have different Latin names based upon the plant from which the essential oil was extracted. The blends in this book have been tested using the essential oils listed in this chart.

Which essential oils treat which ailments?

The table contains information about what each essential oil is effective in treating. This list focuses on the ailments from this book and includes reference from other trained and knowledgeable Aromatherapists. Looking at the "good for" column, and knowing that an essential oil is good for a particular ailment is just a starting point. You also need to know how much of the oil to use, whether you should mix the oil with other essential oils, how you should dilute the blend, how frequently you should use the blend, and what you can expect. The blends in this book include this information; therefore, you can treat your ailment with confidence. If you see recipes or blends on websites, other books, magazine articles, etc., be sure that the recipe was tested by a trained and competent aromatherapy professional.

Are all essential oils safe to use?

The Safety Information column gives you known cautions for some essential oils. In this book, I rarely suggest that you use an essential oil undiluted because they are so concentrated. However, if you choose to use an essential oil undiluted, please use a skin patch test first. To do so, apply a drop of the essential oil on a patch of skin, such as the skin above your elbow on the inside of your arm. Wait 15 minutes; if you have a skin reaction, wash the area immediately with cool water and do not use that essential oil.

If you are pregnant, ALWAYS make sure the oils in a blend are safe for you to use. Also, do not take essential oils internally unless specifically instructed by a certified aromatherapist.

Oil/Latin Name/Source	Good for	Safety Information
Basil Ocimum basilicum Flower and leaves	Antiseptic, Back Pain, Carpal Tunnel, Cellulite, Circulation, Concentration, Cramps, Depression, Digestion, Ear aches, Fever, Headache, Immune System Tonic, Pain, Sinus, Stress, Tension	Should be avoided during pregnancy. Avoid in epileptics. In high concentrations may irritate the skin. Avoid using on children under 12.
Bergamot Citrus bergamia Hybrid of bitter orange and lemon, taken from the peel of the fruit	Acne, Antiseptic, Anxiety, Astringent, Concentration, Coughs, Cramps, Deodorant, Depression, Digestion, Eczema, Expectorant, Fever Reducing, PMS, Psoriasis, Skin Cleanser, Smoking Cessation, Stress	Increases the photosensitivity of the skin, do not use on the skin in sunlight.
Black Pepper Piper nigrum Berries	Analgesic, Antiseptic, Aphrodisiac, Colds, Colic, Constipation, Cramps, Digestion, Fever, Flu, Immune System Stimulant, Pain, Rheumatism, Sprains	In high concentrations may irritate the skin.
Carrot Daucus carota Seeds	Arthritis, Burns, Colic, Cramps, Dermatitis, Eczema, PMS, Psoriasis, Rash, Skin, Sunburn, Wrinkles	Non-toxic, Non-irritant, Non-sensitizing.
Cedarwood Juniperus virginiana Wood	Acne, Anger, Antiseptic, Arthritis, Astringent, Back Pain, Bronchitis, Concentration, Dandruff, Dermatitis, Eczema, Hair Growth, Hair Loss, Immune System Tonic, Inflammation, Insomnia, Rashes, Scalp Health, Sedative, Tension	Should be avoided during pregnancy. In high concentrations may irritate the skin. Avoid using on children under 12.

Oil/Latin Name/Source	Good for	Safety Information
Chamomile Anthemis nobilis (Roman chamomile) Matricaria chamomilla (German chamomile) Flower	Analgesic, Acne, Allergies, Anger, Anti-Inflammatory (German is better), Antiseptic, Anxiety, Arthritis, Back Pain, Bruises, Burns, Children, Colic, Constipation, Cramps, Depression, Dermatitis, Diaper Rash, Ear Infections, Eczema, Fever, Headache, Immune System Tonic, Infections, Inflammation, Insect Bites, Insomnia, Itching, Pain, PMS, Rash, Skin, Sprains, Sunburn, Tension, Throat Infections	Non-toxic, Non-irritant, Non-sensitizing.
Cinnamon Cinnamomum zeylancium Leaves and twigs	Colds, Coughs, Constipation, Flu, Immune System Stimulant, Infections, Rheumatism, Viral Infections, Warts	Avoid during pregnancy. Avoid using on children under 12. May irritate skin.
Clary Sage Salvia sclarea Flower	Acne, Antiseptic, Anxiety, Bronchitis, Burns, Colic, Cramps, Deodorant, Depression, Dermatitis, Headache, Hot Flashes, Inflammation, Insomnia, Pain, PMS, Skin, Stress, Sunburn, Tension, Wrinkles	Avoid in epileptics. Avoid during pregnancy. Avoid if you have estrogen-dependent conditions. Avoid using on children under 12.
Clove Eugenia caryophyllata Leaves and flowers	Antiseptic, Arthritis, Bronchitis, Bruises, Colic, Congestion, Cramps, Digestion, Immune System Stimulant, Inflammation, Insect Repellent, Insomnia, Pain, Sinus, Sprains, Toothache	Avoid during pregnancy. Avoid using on children under 12. May irritate skin.
Cypress Cupressus sempervirens Leaves and twigs	Acne, Antiseptic, Astringent, Athlete's Foot, Bronchitis, Bruises, Carpal Tunnel, Cellulite, Circulation, Coughs, Cramps, Crying, Dandruff, Deodorant, Diaper Rash, Eczema, Hot Flashes, Inflammation, Pain, Sinus, Sprains	Should be avoided during pregnancy.
Eucalyptus Eucalyptus globulus, Eucalyptus citriodora Leaves and branches	Acne, Antiseptic, Arthritis, Asthma, Athlete's Foot, Back Pain, Bronchitis, Carpal Tunnel, Circulation, Colds, Concentration, Congestion, Cough Expectorant, Cramps, Deodorant, Digestion, Ear Aches, Fever, Flu, Headache, Immune System Stimulant, Infections, Inflammation, Insect Bites, Itching, Muscle Pain, Pain, Rash, Rheumatism, Sinus Infection, Sore Throat, Sprains	In high concentrations may irritate the skin.

Oil/Latin Name/Source	Good for	Safety Information
Fennel Foeniculum vulgare Fruit	Cellulite, Colic, Constipation, Cramps, Digestion, Coughs, Overindulgence, PMS, Stress, Wrinkles	Avoid if you have seizure disorders. Avoid during pregnancy. Avoid using on children under 12. Avoid if you have kidney problems.
Frankincense Boswellia thurifera Resin	Antiseptic, Astringent, Bronchitis, Burns, Colds, Congestion, Coughs, Cramps, Dermatitis, Immune System Tonic, Inflammation, Sinus, Sunburn, Stress, Wrinkles	Non-toxic, Non-irritant, Non-sensitizing.
Geranium Pelargonium odorantissimum Flowers	Acne, Antiseptic, Astringent, Anxiety, Athlete's Foot, Bruises, Burns, Cellulite, Depression, Dermatitis, Diaper Rash, Eczema, Hormones, Infections, Inflammation, Insect Repellent, Insomnia, Irritability, Itching, PMS, Skin, Sunburn, Tension, Wrinkles	Avoid if you have low blood sugar.
Ginger Zingiber officinale Root	Arthritis, Back Pain, Bronchitis, Circulation, Colds, Colic, Constipation, Coughs, Cramps, Digestion, Flu, Morning Sickness, Motion Sickness, Muscle Tension, Pain, Rheumatism, Sprains	May irritate skin.
Grapefruit Citrus deucumana Fruit peels	Cellulite, Circulation, Cramps, Depression, Hair, Headache, PMS, Overeating, Skin	Increases photosensitivity of the skin
Juniper Juniperus communis Berries	Acne, Arthritis, Cellulite, Coughs, Dermatitis, Rheumatism	Should be avoided during pregnancy. Do not use if you have kidney problems. Avoid using on children under 12.
Lavender Lavandula officinalus, Lavendula augustofolia Flowers	Acne, Anger, Antiseptic, Anxiety, Athlete's Foot, Bronchitis, Bruises, Burns, Carpal Tunnel, Cellulite, Circulation, Colds, Colic, Cramps, Dandruff, Depression, Dermatitis, Diaper Rash, Digestion, Earaches, Eczema, Flu, Hair Loss, Headache, Infections, Inflammation, Insect Bites, Insomnia, Irritability, Itching, Pain, PMS, Rash, Rheumatism, Sinus, Skin, Sprains, Stress, Sunburn, Wrinkles	Non-toxic, Non-irritant, Non-sensitizing.

Oil/Latin Name/Source	Good for	Safety Information
Lemon Citrus limonum Fruit peels	Acne, Athlete's Foot, Astringent, Blond Hair, Bronchitis, Cellulite, Colds, Concentration, Congestion, Coughs, Cramps, Dandruff, Disinfectant, Fever, Flu, Headache, Immune System Stimulant, Infections, Inflammation, Insect Bites, Rheumatism, Stress, Throat Infections	Increases photosensitivity of the skin.
Lemongrass Cymbopogon citrates Leaves	Antiseptic, Astringent, Back Pain, Bruises, Carpal Tunnel, Circulation, Concentration, Digestion, Fatigue, Grumpiness, Headache, Immune System Stimulant, Inflammation, Insect Bites, Pain	May irritate skin.
Marjoram Origamnum majorana Leaves	Anxiety, Arthritis, Back Pain, Bruises, Carpal Tunnel, Circulation, Colic, Constipation, Cramps, Headache, Insomnia, Muscle Tension, Pain, PMS, Sinuses, Sprains, Stress, Tension	Should be avoided during pregnancy.
Myrrh Commiphora myrrha Bark/resin	Bacterial Infections, Bronchitis, Candida, Dermatitis, Diarrhea, Fungal Infections, Immune System Tonic, Tension, Wounds, Wrinkles	Should be avoided during pregnancy.
Nutmeg Mystica fragrans Seeds and husks	Arthritis, Back Pain, Constipation, Circulation, Depression, Digestion, Immune System Stimulant, Muscle Soreness, Pain, PMS, Rheumatism, Sprains, Stress, Tiredness	Do not with epilepsy. Use moderately during pregnancy.
Orange Citrus aurantium Fruit peels	Anxiety, Cellulite, Concentration, Constipation, Dermatitis, Digestion, Disinfectant, Fever, Inflammation, Insect Repellent, Insomnia, PMS, Skin	Increases photosensitivity of the skin
Patchouli Pogostemon patchouli Leaves	Aphrodisiac, Constipation, Dandruff, Dermatitis, Diaper Rash, Eczema, Immune System Tonic, Inflammation, Moth Repellent, Skin, Viral Infections, Wrinkles, Yeast Infections	Should be avoided during pregnancy.

Oil/Latin Name/ Source	Good for	Safety Information
Peppermint Mentha piperata Leaves	Acne, Antiseptic, Arthritis, Back Pain, Bronchitis, Bruises, Burns, Carpal Tunnel, Circulation, Colds, Colic, Concentration, Congestion, Constipation, Cramps, Dandruff, Dermatitis, Digestion, Earaches, Flu, Headache, Infections, Inflammation, Insect Bites, Itching, Nausea, Pain, Rheumatism, Sinus, Sore Muscles, Sprains, Tension, Vomiting	Not for children under 6 (orally) or in high concentrations. Can be a slight irritant for sensitive skin. Avoid during pregnancy and nursing. May counteract homeopathic treatments.
Pine Pinus Cembra Wood	Antiseptic, Arthritis, Back Pain, Blood Circulation, Bronchitis, Cold, Cramps, Depression, Flu, Hair Loss, Immune System Stimulant, Infections, Muscle Spasm, Rheumatism, Scalp, Sinus, Sprains	Avoid if you have high blood pressure. May irritate skin.
Rosemary Rosmarinus officinalis Leaves and flowers	Acne, Antiseptic, Arthritis, Asthma, Back Pain, Bronchitis, Bruises, Brunette Hair, Burns, Cellulite, Circulation, Colds, Colic, Concentration, Cramps, Dandruff, Dermatitis, Earaches, Eczema, Flu, Headache, Infections, Inflammation, Insect Bites, Pain, Rheumatism, Sinus, Sore Muscles, Sprains, Sunburn, Wrinkles	Do not use during pregnancy or with epilepsy. Avoid if you have high blood pressure.
Rosewood Aniba rosaeodora Wood	Coughs, Depression, Dermatitis, Headaches, Immune System Tonic, Skin, Wrinkles	Non-toxic, Non-irritant, Non-sensitizing.
Sandalwood Santalum album Wood	Acne, Antiseptic, Anxiety, Aphrodisiac, Bronchitis, Cramps, Dermatitis, Immune System Tonic, Inflammation, Insomnia, Sinus, Skin, Stress. Tension, Throat Infection	Not with kidney infections.
Spruce Tsuga Canadensis Bark	Arthritis, Back Pain, Candida, Colds, Hyperthyroidism, Immune System Depression, Pain, Rheumatism	Non-toxic, Non-irritant, Non-sensitizing.
Tangerine Citrus Madurensis Fruit peels	Constipation, Depression, Insomnia, Irritability, PMS, Tension	Increases photosensitivity of the skin

Oil/Latin Name/ Source	Good for	Safety Information
Tea Tree Melaleuca alternifolia Leaves	Acne, Antiviral, Antibacterial, Antiseptic, Athlete's Foot, Bronchitis, Congestion, Coughs, Dandruff, Dermatitis, Earaches, Eczema, Flu, Immune System Stimulant, Infections, Inflammation, Insect Bites, Itching, Rash, Sinus, Yeast Infections	Non-toxic, Non-irritant, Non-sensitizing.
Thyme Thymus vulgaris Leaves and flowers	Antibacterial, Antiviral, Arthritis, Athlete's Foot, Back Pain, Bronchitis, Bruises, Cellulite, Concentration, Colds, Congestion, Coughs, Cramps, Dandruff, Dermatitis, Earaches, Eczema, Flu, Eczema, Infections, Insect Bites, Pain, Sinus, Sprains, Tiredness	Do not use undiluted, in pregnancy, for epilepsy, on children, for high blood pressure.
Vetiver Vetivaria zizanoides Roots	Antiseptic, Aphrodisiac, Arthritis, Back Pain, Depression, Immune System Stimulant, Insomnia, Muscle Relaxant, Pain, Rheumatism, Skin, Sprains, Stress, Tension	Non-toxic, Non-irritant, Non-sensitizing.
Yarrow Achillea millefolium Herb	Arthritis, Constipation, Cramps, Diaper Rash, Eczema, Immune System Tonic, Inflammation, Scars, Wounds	Non-toxic, Non-irritant, Non-sensitizing.
Ylang Ylang Canangium odoratum Flowers	Anger, Antiseptic, Aphrodisiac, Circulation, Cramps, Depression, Fever, Immune System Tonic, Irritability, Pain, PMS, Skin, Tension	Avoid if you have a headache or nausea.

Bibliography for information in the Essential Oil Chart:

Complete Aromatherapy Handbook, Suzanne Fischer-Rizzi, c 1990, Sterling Publishing Company

The Complete Book of Essential Oils & Aromatherapy, Valerie Ann Worwood, c 1991, New World Library

The Art of Aromatherapy, Robert B. Tisserand, c 1977, Healing Arts Press

The Encyclopaedia of Essential Oils, Julia Lawless c1992, Element Books Limited

Ordering Essential Oils

All the essential oils are listed on the order form on the next page.

Step 1:   **Determine which Essential Oils you want to purchase.**

Step 2:   **Determine which size bottle you want to purchase.**

.5 fluid ounces = approximately 380 drops

.25 fluid ounces = approximately 190 drops

.125 fluid ounces = approximately 95 drops

Note: Don't order more than you plan to use within the next 6 months. While I offer fresh quality oils, the shelf life of essential oils is about 18 months.

Step 3:   **Order the correct number and size of dropper caps.**

Step 4:   **Determine the appropriate shipping and handling fee.**

Up to 8 bottles = $5.00

Up to 16 bottles = $8.00

More than 16 bottles = $12.00

Step 5:   If you want the oils shipped to a different address, please add a note with that address.

Step 6:   **Send check or money order to:**

Judith Fitzsimmons

2276 Henpeck Lane

Franklin, TN 37064

NOTE: Please go to www.aromatherapysolutions.com to verify my address!

Therapeutic Grade, High Quality Essential Oils at Wholesale Prices

Oil	Size	Price *	Qty	Size	Price *	Qty	Size	Price *	Qty
Basil	0.125	$1.50		0.25	$2.25		0.5	$3.50	
Bergamot	0.125	$1.50		0.25	$3.00		0.5	$5.00	
Black Pepper	0.125	$1.50		0.25	$2.25		0.5	$3.50	
Carrot	0.125	$3.00		0.25	$5.00		0.5	$9.00	
Cedarwood	0.125	$1.50		0.25	$2.25		0.5	$3.50	
Chamomile	0.125	$10.00		0.25	$20.00		0.5	$30.00	
Cinnamon	0.125	$1.50		0.25	$2.25		0.5	$3.50	
Clary Sage	0.125	$2.50		0.25	$4.00		0.5	$6.00	
Clove	0.125	$1.50		0.25	$2.25		0.5	$3.50	
Cypress	0.125	$1.50		0.25	$3.00		0.5	$5.00	
Eucalyptus	0.125	$1.50		0.25	$2.25		0.5	$3.50	
Fennel	0.125	$1.50		0.25	$2.25		0.5	$3.50	
Frankincense	0.125	$4.00		0.25	$7.00		0.5	$12.00	
Geranium	0.125	$2.50		0.25	$4.00		0.5	$6.00	
Ginger	0.125	$1.50		0.25	$2.25		0.5	$3.50	
Grapefruit	0.125	$1.50		0.25	$2.25		0.5	$3.50	
Juniper	0.125	$2.50		0.25	$4.00		0.5	$6.00	
Lavender	0.125	$3.00		0.25	$5.00		0.5	$9.00	
Lemon	0.125	$1.50		0.25	$2.00		0.5	$3.50	
Lemongrass	0.125	$1.50		0.25	$2.25		0.5	$3.50	
Marjoram	0.125	$1.50		0.25	$3.00		0.5	$5.00	
Myrrh	0.125	$7.00		0.25	$12.00		0.5	$20.00	
Nutmeg	0.125	$1.50		0.25	$3.00		0.5	$5.00	
Orange	0.125	$1.50		0.25	$2.25		0.5	$3.50	
Patchouli	0.125	$1.50		0.25	$2.25		0.5	$3.50	
Peppermint	0.125	$1.50		0.25	$2.25		0.5	$3.50	
Pine	0.125	$1.50		0.25	$2.25		0.5	$3.50	
Rosemary	0.125	$1.50		0.25	$2.25		0.5	$3.50	
Rosewood	0.125	$1.50		0.25	$3.00		0.5	$5.00	
Sandalwood	0.125	$7.00		0.25	$12.00		0.5	$20.00	
Spruce	0.125	$1.50		0.25	$2.25		0.5	$3.50	
Tangerine	0.125	$1.50		0.25	$2.25		0.5	$3.50	
Tea Tree	0.125	$1.50		0.25	$2.25		0.5	$3.50	
Thyme	0.125	$1.50		0.25	$3.00		0.5	$5.00	
Vetiver	0.125	$2.50		0.25	$4.00		0.5	$6.00	
Yarrow	0.125	$9.00		0.25	$15.00		0.5	$26.00	
Ylang Ylang	0.125	$3.00		0.25	$5.00		0.5	$9.00	
* Prices subject to change without notice									
DROPPERS	0.125	$.50		0.25	$.50		0.5	$.50	
Name									
Address									
Phone									
Email									

Index

B

Baby Blues 131. See also Depression, Postpartum Depression
Baby Blues Soother 132, 133
Back Pain 1, 15, 16, 17, 18, 278, 279, 280, 281, 282, 283
Back Pain Relief 16, 17
Back Pain Soother 17, 18
Back Pain Support 18
Bag Balm 59
Bases 270, 274. See also Carrier Oils
Basil 16, 20, 25, 43, 94, 103, 104, 172, 181, 184, 244, 246, 262, 278, 285
Bedtime 18, 32, 55, 88, 149, 150, 258, 259, 260. See also Insomnia
Bergamot 69, 70, 94, 95, 96, 98, 100, 103, 109, 113, 116, 120, 121, 125, 126, 127, 131, 134, 136, 137, 162, 190, 262, 264, 265, 278, 285
Big Relief for Little Kids 225
Birch 9
Bircher Muesli 160
Black and Blue 202. See also Bruises
Black Pepper 4, 9, 10, 13, 25, 31, 35, 37, 39, 124, 127, 158, 184, 202, 204, 248, 278, 285
Blemish 49, 50. See also Acne
Blemish Blocker 49, 50
Boo-boos 209. See also Wounds
Borage Oil 272. See also Carrier Oils
Borage Seed 75, 77, 167, 168, 241. See also Carrier Oils
Bronchitis 139, 141, 142, 144, 145, 278, 279, 280, 281, 282, 283
Bronchitis, acute 142
Bronchitis, chronic 142
Bronchitis Blaster 144, 145
Bruise Assistance 204
Bruise Reducer 202, 203
Bruise Soother 203, 204
Bugs Away 222
Burn 205. See also Burns
Burn, first degree 206
Burn, second degree 206
Burn, third degree 206
Burn Relief 207, 208
Burn Soother 207
Burns 48, 200, 205, 206, 217, 272, 275, 278, 279, 280, 282

C

Calm and Heal 230, 231
Camellia Oil 272

Cardamom 103
Carpal Tunnel Relief 20, 21
Carpal Tunnel Soother 21, 22
Carpal Tunnel Syndrome 1, 19, 20
Carrier Oils 5, 6, 10, 11, 12, 13, 14, 17, 18, 21, 22, 26, 27, 30, 31, 33, 36, 37,
    41, 44, 45, 46, 55, 56, 57, 60, 65, 66, 70, 71, 72, 75, 76, 77, 78, 84, 87,
    88, 95, 96, 97, 98, 99, 100, 101, 105, 106, 110, 111, 116, 117, 118, 121,
    122, 128, 129, 133, 134, 144, 145, 155, 156, 159, 160, 163, 182, 185,
    186, 189, 190, 193, 196, 199, 203, 204, 211, 215, 218, 219, 223, 224,
    225, 239, 240, 245, 246, 249, 252, 254, 263, 264, 265, 271
Carrot 9, 54, 59, 60, 61, 69, 74, 75, 77, 80, 81, 83, 84, 86, 89, 168, 206, 233,
    248, 262, 278, 285
Cedar xv, 54, 109, 138
Cedarwood 9, 16, 56, 57, 61, 64, 94, 95, 103, 105, 124, 127, 131, 133, 136, 143,
    166, 167, 169, 170, 184, 217, 256, 258, 259, 278, 285
Cellulite 235, 243, 244, 275, 278, 279, 280, 281, 282, 283
Chamomile xv, 4, 9, 10, 12, 14, 16, 17, 25, 26, 30, 33, 35, 39, 40, 41, 49, 52, 54,
    55, 56, 57, 59, 60, 62, 64, 65, 66, 69, 71, 72, 74, 80, 83, 84, 94, 96, 97,
    98, 100, 108, 113, 118, 120, 121, 125, 129, 131, 136, 138, 158, 160, 162,
    163, 164, 172, 174, 181, 182, 184, 186, 189, 202, 203, 206, 207, 208,
    210, 211, 217, 218, 219, 222, 224, 225, 226, 228, 229, 230, 231, 233,
    234, 248, 249, 251, 252, 253, 256, 258, 259, 260, 262, 263, 266, 270,
    279, 285
Chapped Hands Cure 62
Child 149
Child and Youngster Cold Relief 149
Children's Rash Treatment 70
Cider Vinegar 81, 82
Cinnamon 145, 156, 158, 176, 184, 185, 213, 215, 279, 285
Clary Sage 17, 25, 28, 33, 49, 52, 54, 59, 61, 86, 88, 94, 96, 98, 108, 113, 114,
    118, 120, 121, 125, 129, 131, 134, 136, 137, 170, 181, 182, 206, 217,
    233, 248, 256, 257, 258, 259, 260, 262, 264, 265, 266, 279, 285
Clove 4, 5, 9, 14, 25, 26, 30, 35, 39, 41, 143, 144, 145, 153, 154, 155, 184, 185,
    188, 192, 202, 203, 204, 217, 218, 248, 279, 285
Cluster Headache 180. See also Headaches
Coconut Oil 272. See also Carrier Oils
Colds 139, 149, 150, 278, 279, 280, 281, 282, 283
Colic Relief 248, 249
Colic Soother 249
Common Colds 147. See also Colds
Compression 3
Concentration 90, 102, 104, 278, 279, 281, 282, 283
Concentration Room Spray 104
Congestion Relief 154, 155
Congestion Soother 155, 156

D

G

H

Hair Rinse 168
Hair Rinse for Dandruff 168
Hazelnut Oil 259, 273. See also Carrier Oils
Headache, cluster 180
Headache, migraine 180
Headache, sinus 180
Headache, tension 180
Headache Relief 181, 182
Headache Soother 182
Heartburn 188. See also Indigestion
Helplessness 108. See also Depression, Postpartum Depression
House Cleaner 194, 197, 198

I

Immune System 139, 183, 185, 186, 278, 279, 280, 281, 282, 283
Immune System Stimulant 185, 186, 278, 279, 281, 282, 283
Immune System Stimulant – Children 186
Immune System Stimulant – Teens and Adults 185
Immune System Tonic 186, 278, 279, 280, 281, 282, 283
Indigestion xxiv, 140, 187, 188, 190
Indigestion Comforter 190
Indigestion Soother 189, 190
Infant Earache Relief 172, 173
Infection xxi, 177, 200, 212, 214, 215, 279, 282
Infection Relief 214, 215
Inflammation 8, 200, 216, 217, 218, 219, 275, 278, 279, 280, 281, 282, 283
Inflammation, acute 217
Inflammation, chronic 217
Inflammation Relief 218
Inflammation Soother 218, 219
Insects 220
Insect Bites 200, 217, 224, 225, 279, 280, 281, 282, 283
Insect Bites Relief 224, 225
Insect Repellent 223, 279, 280, 281
Insomnia 235, 255, 257, 258, 259, 278, 279, 280, 281, 282, 283
Insomnia Bath 259
Insomnia Body Rub 257, 258, 259
Insomnia Relief 257
Intense Indigestion Relief 189
Irritability 91, 123, 125, 127, 128, 129, 280, 282, 283
Irritability Relief 128, 129
Irritability Relief – Option 1 128
Irritability Relief – Option 2 129
Irritating Indigestion Soother 189, 190

Itching 200, 217, 227, 236, 275, 279, 280, 282, 283

J

Jojoba Oil 273. See also Carrier Oils
Juniper xv, 9, 10, 33, 49, 54, 94, 99, 106, 120, 122, 189, 244, 245, 246, 262, 280, 285

K

Kid's Sinus Treatment 198. See also Carrier Oils
Kukui Nut Oil 273

L

Ladies Preferred Sinus Treatment 196
Lavender xv, 4, 5, 6, 11, 13, 17, 18, 20, 21, 25, 26, 29, 31, 33, 35, 36, 37, 39, 40, 43, 44, 49, 50, 51, 52, 54, 55, 56, 57, 59, 60, 61, 64, 66, 69, 70, 71, 72, 74, 75, 76, 77, 78, 80, 81, 82, 83, 84, 86, 87, 88, 89, 94, 97, 100, 101, 104, 105, 106, 110, 113, 114, 115, 120, 121, 122, 124, 125, 126, 128, 129, 136, 137, 138, 143, 146, 148, 149, 151, 154, 163, 164, 166, 167, 168, 169, 170, 172, 173, 174, 176, 177, 178, 181, 182, 188, 189, 192, 199, 202, 204, 206, 207, 208, 210, 211, 213, 214, 217, 218, 219, 222, 223, 224, 225, 226, 228, 230, 231, 233, 234, 238, 239, 240, 241, 242, 244, 248, 249, 251, 252, 253, 254, 256, 257, 258, 260, 262, 263, 266, 280, 285
Lemon 25, 29, 40, 49, 50, 51, 80, 81, 82, 83, 89, 94, 97, 103, 105, 106, 110, 111, 113, 114, 115, 120, 122, 124, 126, 136, 138, 143, 144, 153, 154, 155, 160, 162, 166, 168, 169, 176, 177, 178, 181, 182, 184, 186, 190, 213, 214, 215, 238, 240, 241, 244, 245, 246, 260, 281, 285
Lemongrass 16, 20, 21, 22, 25, 43, 45, 46, 103, 181, 184, 222, 223, 229, 281, 285
Lethargy 91, 112, 113, 115, 116
Lethargy Treatment 116

M

Macadamia Nut Oil 273. See also Carrier Oils
Man's Man Sinus Treatment 193
Mandarin 94
Marjoram 4, 9, 11, 13, 16, 18, 20, 21, 22, 25, 27, 28, 31, 33, 35, 36, 39, 43, 46, 94, 99, 101, 109, 113, 125, 131, 136, 158, 181, 182, 202, 204, 248, 256, 262, 276, 281, 285
Massage Away Stress 137, 138
Migraine 180. See also Headaches

Osteo Arthritis 8. See also Arthritis

P

Pain 1, 38, 39, 40, 41, 42, 179, 278, 279, 280, 281, 282, 283
Pain, acute 39
Pain, chronic 39
Pain Management 13
Pain Relief 1, 38, 39, 40
Pain Reliever 40
Pain Relieving 189
Pain Soother 40, 41
Palma Rosa 158, 262
Panic 90, 92, 93, 94, 99, 100, 101
Panic Relief 100, 101
Panic Relief – Option 1 100
Panic Relief – Option 2 101
Parsley 248
Patchouli 54, 56, 59, 62, 64, 66, 74, 80, 82, 86, 94, 108, 125, 128, 131, 158,
        160, 166, 184, 186, 217, 231, 239, 251, 254, 281, 285
Peanut Oil 273, 275. See also Carrier Oils
Pecan Oil 274. See also Carrier Oils
Peppermint 4, 6, 9, 10, 12, 13, 16, 17, 18, 20, 21, 22, 25, 29, 32, 35, 36, 37, 39,
        40, 43, 44, 45, 49, 54, 55, 71, 103, 106, 113, 124, 125, 126, 143, 144,
        150, 151, 153, 156, 158, 159, 166, 172, 174, 176, 177, 181, 182, 188,
        189, 190, 192, 196, 202, 203, 204, 206, 207, 208, 217, 219, 222, 223,
        224, 225, 228, 229, 231, 234, 242, 248, 282, 285
Perimenopausal 20
Personal Concentration Blend 104, 105
Photosensitivity 278, 280, 281, 282
Pimples 48. See also Acne
Pine 4, 9, 16, 25, 124, 148, 185, 192, 193, 199, 213, 282, 285
PMS 131, 261, 262, 263, 264, 265, 278, 279, 280, 281, 282, 283
PMS, cramps 261
PMS Lifter 265
PMS Relief for Grumps 264, 265
PMS Relief for Tension 263, 264
PMS Soother 263
PMS Uplifter 264
Poison Ivy 200, 217, 227, 228, 229, 230
Poison Ivy Relief 228, 229
Poison Ivy Soother 229, 230
Postpartum Depression 91, 130, 133, 134
Postpartum Depression Relief 133, 134
Preferred Sinus Treatment 195

R

S

T

V

W

Y

Z

About the Author

Judith Fitzsimmons, the author of *"Seasons of Aromatherapy"* has over 15 years experience as a certified aromatherapist helping people at all stages of life through "Aromatherapy Solutions", an aromatherapy blending business found on the web at www.aromatherapysolutions.com.

She balances her life as a businesswoman, author, and speaker with being the mother of a beautiful and active 12-year-old daughter, Chelsea. These activities enhance her life and her work. Over the years Judith has focused her work on formulating and developing blends for the common ailments that people of all ages deal with. Judith's second book, *"Aromatherapy Answers"* provides the answers to the ailments.

Along with Chelsea, Judith shares her life with her fiancé Mark, and their dogs, Cooper and Rusty in Williamson County, Tennessee.

About the Coauthor

Paula M. Bousquet, coauthor of *"Seasons of Aromatherapy"* has been a writer and editor for over 20 years. An avid herb gardener, her day job is as a medical writer for Pfizer, Inc.